SEEING IS BELIEVING: A QUANTITATIVE STUDY OF POSTHYPNOTIC SUGGESTION AND THE ALTERING OF SUBCONSCIOUS BELIEFS TO ENHANCE VISUAL CAPABILITIES INCLUDING THE POTENTIAL FOR NONPHYSICAL SIGHT

by

Joseph Sansone

A dissertation submitted

in partial fulfillment of the requirements

for the degree of Doctor of Philosophy

in Psychology with a concentration in Transpersonal Psychology

Sofia University

Palo Alto, California

August 2, 2019

I certify that I have read and approved the content and presentation of this dissertation:

_____   _____
Marilyn Schlitz, Ph.D., Committee Chairperson   Date

_____   _____
Angel Morgan, Ph.D., Committee Member   Date

_____   _____
John Elfers, Ph.D., Committee Member   Date

Copyright

©

Joseph Sansone

2019

All Rights Reserved

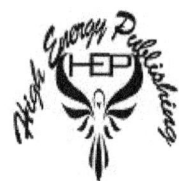

Fort Myers, FL
ISBN # 978-0-578-59557-3
Library of Congress Control Number:2019916654

Abstract

Seeing is Believing: A Quantitative Study of Posthypnotic Suggestion and the Altering of Subconscious Beliefs to Enhance Visual Capabilities Including the Potential for Nonphysical Sight

by

Joseph Sansone

This quantitative study used posthypnotic suggestion to measure for improvements in visual capabilities utilizing standard eye charts. Participants' vision was tested prior to hypnosis with a standard eye chart adjacent to participants. Participants were hypnotized and given a posthypnotic suggestion to enhance vision. Participants' vision was tested again using a different variation of a standard eye chart to measure for visual improvement. Participants were hypnotized again. While hypnotized, a dry-erase board was placed in front of a single-line eye chart of 5 letters, obstructing all lines of sight to the eye chart. Participants were given a posthypnotic suggestion inducing a negative hallucination rendering the dry-erase whiteboard that was obstructing the line of sight to the eye chart invisible, and were provided suggestions to see through or around the obstruction. Conscious amnesia of the posthypnotic suggestion was embedded in the suggestion rendering the negative hallucination of the object of obstruction unavailable to conscious awareness. Participants were then tested again using a single-line eye chart of 5 letters. A total of 50 participants were selected for the study on visual enhancement and a subset of 5 participants capable of a negative hallucination were tested to explore the potential for nonphysical sight. Participants were debriefed that deception was used in the experiment. Results were statistically significant for eyesight improvement. Results were also statistically significant for evidence of nonphysical sight, although considered preliminary due to a small sample size. Implications of the findings are discussed.

Dedication

Dedicated to my father

A disabled combat veteran of the Korean Conflict who was awarded a combat infantry badge,

received the bronze and silver star as well as a unit citation for his services.

He taught me the power of the human mind.

Acknowledgments

I would like to acknowledge my dissertation committee for their willingness to support unconventional research; also, my extraordinary hypnosis instructors who taught me the lost healing art of hypnosis back in 1997; and my wife and family for their support. Special thanks to those that assisted me during the research and to those willing participants who made this research possible.

Table of Contents

Abstract iii

Dedication v

Acknowledgments vi

List of Tables xi

List of Figures xii

Chapter 1: Introduction 1

    The Roots of Hypnosis as a Healing Modality 1

        Defining or describing hypnosis and related terms. 3

        Subconscious mind and subconscious beliefs. 6

    Specific Research Questions and Hypothesis 8

    Personal Significance 9

    Purpose, Significance, and Importance of the Study 10

    Study Design 11

    Organization of the Study 11

Chapter 2: Literature Review 12

    Hypnosis and Mind-body Healing 12

        Hypnosis and pain. 12

        Hypnosis mental health benefits. 15

        Hypnosis, headaches, and tinnitus. 18

        Hypnosis and sleep. 19

        Hypnosis, arthritis, sickle cell anemia, and Parkinson's. 20

        Hypnosis and changes in the brain. 21

        Hypnosis and childbirth. 22

        Hypnosis and stroke recovery. 23

        Hypnosis and surgery. 24

        Hypnosis and regeneration. 25

        Hypnosis and blood flow. 26

        Hypnosis, diabetes, alopecia, and skin disorders. 26

        Hypnosis, asthma, and allergies. 27

        Hypnosis and bowel disorders. 28

        Hypnosis and immune system enhancement. 28

        Hypnosis and performance. 29

        Hypnosis and vision. 30

    Parapsychological Research 32

        Hypnosis and psi/ESP phenomena. 32

        Neurobiological model for psi. 34

        Morphic fields and morphic resonance. 34

    Conclusion and Rationale for This Study 37

Chapter 3: Research Method 39

    Rationale for Selecting Design 40

    Description of Research Design 40

    Instruments of Measurement/Measurement Techniques 41

    Previous Research and the Uniqueness of This Study 41

    Participants 42

    Materials 43

    Procedure 43

  Informed consent. 43

  Specific interventions.. 44

  Statistical analysis. 47

  Ethical consideration.. 47

 Limitations of the Study.. 49

 Issues of Internal/External Validity 50

Chapter 4: Results 53

 Nonphysical Sight... 53

  Nonphysical sight among L6 participants.. 54

  Nonphysical sight among non-L6 participants. 56

  Nonphysical sight among L6 and non-L6 participants combined. 56

  Between-group comparison of nonphysical sight among L6 versus non-L6 participants. 56

 Posthypnotic Enhancement of Visual Accuracy 58

Chapter 5: Discussion 62

 Hypnosis and Visual Acuity 62

  Findings and observations.. 62

  Theories explaining effect.. 64

  Future research. 66

  Potential application... 67

 Hypnosis and Nonphysical Sight 67

  Findings and observations.. 68

  Theories explaining the effect.. 71

   Future research. 73

    Potential applications. 74

  Conclusion 74

References 76

Appendix A: Informed Consent 93

Appendix B: Questionnaire 96

Appendix C: Email Solicitation 97

Appendix D: Chairs in Private Practice Office 98

Appendix E: Eye Chart Assessments 100

Appendix F: Eye Chart on Stand 103

Appendix G: Shielding Eye Chart 105

Appendix H: Shielded Eye Chart 107

Appendix I: Posthypnotic Suggestion Sample 109

List of Tables

Table		Page
1.	Chance and Achieved Accuracy on the Nonphysical Vision Test in the L6 Sample, Non-L6 Sample, and Combined Samples With Results of z-Tests for Sample Proportions	54
2.	Chance and Achieved Accuracy on the Nonphysical Vision Test in the L6 Sample and Non-L6 Sample and Results of a z-Test Comparison of Two Independent Proportions	57
3.	Visual Acuity Before and Following Posthypnotic Visual Enhancement With Results of Within-Subjects t-Test	58

List of Figures

Figure   Page

1. Mean visual acuity before and after posthypnotic enhancement. Error bars represent 95% confidence intervals for population means. 59

2. A frequency histogram showing the distribution of T2–T1 difference scores. 60

Chapter 1: Introduction

This study examined the impact of hypnosis, hypnotic suggestion, and their potential influence of mind-body interactions as well as human potential in the form of *psi* or extra sensory perception (ESP). *Psi* is the first Greek letter in the word *psyche*, which means mind-soul (Lexico, n.d.) and is often used to represent the unknown factor in ESP that cannot be explained by current scientific explanations. For the purposes of this study, the use of the terms psi and ESP are interchangeable. The altering of subconscious beliefs via hypnosis was considered as a potential means to create a mind-body effect and a more direct psi effect. Hypnosis was considered a well-suited vehicle for this research study because, as shall be seen, it is an effective means for altering subconscious beliefs. Evidence that the alteration of subconscious beliefs creates a mind-body healing effect, as well as altering perceptions and assisting an ESP effect, will be presented.

The Roots of Hypnosis as a Healing Modality

Hypnosis was one of the progenitors of Western medicine. According to Machovec (1979), the ancient Greek cult of Asklipios lasted a thousand years. It predated Christianity, was widespread through the Mediterranean, and lasted to around 300 years after the birth of Christ. Hippocrates, often referred to as the father of modern medicine, was an Asklipian physician priest. The caduceus, symbol of the medical profession with two intertwined snakes, dates back to the cult of Asklipios. Machovec wrote that Asklipios was a kind and gentle sleep god. Rather than an imaginary induction, inducing an altered state and followed by suggestions and imagery, the ancient hypnosis session was purportedly acted out in temples over a period of days. Priests appeared at night to patients while they were in a dream-like state and offered them healing suggestions. Seven stages in this ritualistic healing process parallel aspects of the modern hypnosis session. These were change of environment, cleansing or specialness, sacrifice or commitment, repetition, belief in the method, focused attention, and emotional impact (Machovec, 1979). The full scope of knowledge of the Asklipian physician priests is unclear, as is the total measure of interaction with patients, but it is believed that they conducted activities ranging from administration duties to surgeries to mind therapy (Burnett, 2015).

These dream healings, although apparently widely in use, were not without criticism, as Aristotle considered the idea that an actual god would visit a mortal in a dream preposterous (Kool, 2015). According to Hart (1965), these dream visits occurred only after suitable hypnotic conditioning. These dream visits by Asklipios, or more likely the physician priests, often had a healing effect (Gruner, 2010). Although attributed with divine power, these actions of Asklipios at times appeared more like a doctor than a god (Panagiotidou, 2016). Once darkness fell, the physician priests reportedly moved through the temple area performing ceremonies using touch, and sometimes sacred dogs or serpents. The god then appeared to patients giving advice and making incisions that healed by morning. The advice from the priests often regarded diet, exercise, herbal treatments, as well as hygiene. The priests then interpreted the advice in the morning. Patients were then asked to write the positive results they experienced, which would be viewed by newcomers to the temple. This treatment used faith and auto-suggestion through the process of the healing ritual (Retief & Cilliers, 2008).

In modern hypnosis, two basic Ericksonian techniques are presupposition and utilization (James, Flores, & Schober, 2016). Presuppositions are the use of assumptions to create the context for indirect suggestions. Utilization is basically using whatever the hypnotized person brings forth to increase trance or the effect of suggestions. It appears that presupposition was used through the preparation process for the temple healing, as patients received suggestions for healing in multiple forms and even read inscriptions of people that were healed before. Thus, an assumption or expectation was created not only that a healing would occur during the dream state, but that a dream state would be achieved. It also appears that utilization was used after the dream state, during which ostensible messages from the god were interpreted by the priest. Stated differently, whatever the patient dreamed up was likely used to increase a healing effect at the suggestion of the priest. The reported specificity of the advice given during the dream state and consistent themes regarding such advice appears to support the assertion that Asklipian physician priests at least occasionally provided such advice to patients in a trance or a sleeplike state. It would appear that suggestion was used throughout the healing process, before, during, and after the dream healings.

Practicing in the United Kingdom, James Braid (1843) first presented the term *hypnotism*. The Scottish surgeon, at first a skeptical inquirer of mesmerism and animal magnetism, applied the rigors of science to mesmerism. Braid recognized the ability of thought and suggestion under hypnosis to create physiological changes and potentially heal certain conditions and diseases. Braid was aware of the connection between hypnotism and control of the imagination and changes in the body. Emile Coué (1922) expounded on both the imagination and the power of suggestion. He separated the imagination from the will and claimed that the imagination is stronger than the will. He also asserted that the power of suggestion is always at work through the activity of thought and imagination. Notably, self-hypnosis and auto-suggestion were advocated as a healing modality (Coué, 1922). While hypnosis has been in use for at least a couple hundred years, defining it is no simple task.

Defining or describing hypnosis and related terms. According to the American Psychological Association Division 30, hypnosis is defined as "a state of consciousness involving focused attention and reduced peripheral awareness, characterized by an enhanced capacity for response to suggestion" (Elkins, Barabasz, Council, & Spiegel, 2015, p. 382). The new definition is concise and appears to leave open the possibility of multiple theories to explain hypnosis. After decades of debate, the new definition appears to acknowledge the state theory of hypnosis, which is the assertion that the hypnotic trance is an altered state of consciousness (Barabasz & Barabasz, 2015). Others have criticized this new definition as being too concise and creating more concerns rather than less by being too parsimonious, potentially hampering the empirically supported reemerging field of hypnosis, and also for not remaining neutral on the state theory of hypnosis (Lynn et al., 2015). The state theory of hypnosis is that hypnosis is a unique and distinct altered state of consciousness that acts as a kind of incubator to heightened suggestibility, and that this trance or altered state is best created by an induction procedure (Kirsch & Lynn, 1995). The cognitive behavioral therapy theory in hypnosis asserts that hypnotic suggestions are effective because the recipient agrees with the overall purpose and content of the suggestions (Barber & Wilson, 1977).

Hypnotherapy is defined as "the use of hypnosis in the treatment of a medical or psychological disorder or concern" (Elkins et al., 2015, p. 7). Hypnotizability is defined as "an individual's ability to experience suggested alterations in physiology, sensations, emotions, thoughts, or behavior during hypnosis" (Elkins et al., 2015, p. 6). The parsimony with the term *hypnotherapy* may lead to practical problems with the use of the term *psychological* among licensed practitioners who are not licensed psychologists. Beyond that, it should be noted that older phrases such as *hypnotic susceptibility* may be used at times instead of *hypnotizability* in this research when citing studies where that term was used by the researchers.

There are some characteristics attributed to hypnosis that appear supportive of the state theory of hypnosis. Hoeft et al. (2012) think that they may be close to providing a brain signature for hypnosis. Hypnotizability may be related to altered connectivity between the left dorsolateral prefrontal cortex as well as the salience network. The dorsal anterior cingulate cortex, amygdala, anterior insula, and ventral stratum comprise the salience network. The interaction of the executive function areas of the brain and the salience network, rather than brain structure, is the determinant to hypnotizability. These are areas of the brain associated with higher brain functioning and thoughts and emotional regulation, as well as somatic and autonomic functioning. Essentially, this interaction involves multiple areas of the brain, including frontal areas, mid, and hind areas; there is a connectivity between the higher thought processing and emotional, somatic, and autonomic functions of the brain. Researchers have asserted that cognitive style, not brain anatomy, is a salient factor to hypnotizability (Hoeft et al., 2012).

The alpha brain wave frequency is often associated with the commonly referred to state of daydreaming. The theta brain wave frequency exists between the alpha state and the delta state, which is sleep. EEG data demonstrated hypnosis at the alpha and theta frequencies (Halsband, Mueller, Hinterberger, & Strickner, 2009). There is some evidence that theta wave activity is associated with relaxation and alpha waves are associated with susceptibility to suggestion (Williams & Gruzelier, 2001). Higher hypnotic susceptibility may be attributed to increased theta wave activity in the anterior temporal lobe (Elahi, Boostani, & Motie Nasrabadi, 2012). Decreased brain activity in the anterior region of the default mode network may contribute to greater hypnotic susceptibility (McGeown, Mazzoni, Venneri, & Kirsch, 2009). Increased theta wave activity in the parietal and occipital parts of the brain may also be associated with higher hypnotic susceptibility (Freeman, Barabasz, Barabasz, & Warner, 2000).

A posthypnotic suggestion is a suggestion designed to work after the hypnosis session has ended. Posthypnotic suggestion may reduce activity in the anterior cingulate cortex as well as parts of the brain associated with visual activity (Raz, Fan, & Posner, 2005). It should be noted that this study dealt with eliminating the Stroop interference, which involves visual processes, particularly the delayed response when reading words of a color that are printed in another color; for example, the word *red* may be printed in blue. It is reasonable to consider the possibility that the areas of the brain and the ensuing activity may vary with the type of posthypnotic suggestion given.

It may be that hypnosis will never be truly defined. The purpose of providing some empirical descriptive features of hypnosis in this research is to relay that the state of hypnosis and hypnotic suggestion have been demonstrated to create changes in brain activity. This may be connected to ESP.

Subconscious mind and subconscious beliefs. It can be argued that a person has only one mind; however, a distinction between the conscious and subconscious mind is useful and practical. The term subconscious is often used interchangeably with unconscious. Rezaeei and Farahian (2015) reported that there is dispute regarding scholarly definitions of the term unconscious; some scholars consider it a state of a total lack of awareness and others, like Freud, had considered it a repository of memories. Most scholarly and unscholarly definitions of subconscious mind seem to assert that it exists below consciousness, and there is also evidence of subconscious learning in language acquisition (e.g., Rezaeei & Farahian, 2015). The term subconscious rather than unconscious is used regarding subconscious mind and subconscious beliefs because it is more accurate. The prefix *un* means not, whereas the prefix *sub* means below (Merriam-Webster, n.d.). When speaking to the issue of subconscious mind or subconscious beliefs, it is inferred that a region of mind exists below the conscious mind and that there are beliefs that exist below conscious beliefs. Below, in this context, means below or beyond the screen of conscious awareness.

Braid (1843) appears to have used the terms soul and mind interchangeably and described it as nonmaterial consciousness. Braid thought that the soul or mind was separate from the brain, and that the mind or soul and the brain interacted with each other in the same way that the musician and the music were distinct. The mind could affect matter, and matter could affect the mind. He also proposed that the organism is a manifestation of mind or the life principle. He appears to argue that the greater degree of abstraction of mind, the closer to divinity (Braid, 1843). Similarly, William James (1902) recognized the legitimacy of altered states of consciousness and viewed the subconscious mind as a potential interface with God or spiritual or metaphysical reality. Approximately 300 years after the death of Julius Caesar, Plotinus provided a detailed philosophical framework that appears to be the basis of later conceptions of soul or mind interacting with and dispersed through the body. Plotinus (1991) described the One, the Intellectual Principle, and the soul, and told us that the soul gives life to the body. Thus, the idea of a nestled hierarchy of mind spanning from the physical to the divine has a long philosophical history, as does the idea that mind can affect the body.

More recent evidence of the separation of the mind from the brain is exemplified by studies of near-death experiences (Baruss & Mossbridge, 2017). There is also credible evidence of potential nonphysical sight among blind people who have had near-death experiences, which supports the assertion that the mind is separate from the brain (Ring & Cooper, 2008). Once it is considered that the body may actually be an aspect of mind, the possibility that thoughts may alter the body and human capabilities appears a more reasonable proposition. Carter (2010) presented data from the field of quantum physics, including several interpretations of the collapse of the wave function. The collapse of the wave function is the collapsing of a wave particle into either a wave or a particle. The most notable interpretation relevant to this discussion is that the observation of consciousness determines if the wave particle collapses into either a particle or a wave (Carter, 2010). This presents the possibility that mind is present in and guides the formation of matter, and thus leaves open that possibility that mind may alter body.

This separation of the mind from the brain and consideration that mind is present in matter is relevant to this study. It created a framework or reference point that allowed the consideration of a paradigm of reality proposing that a region of mind exists beyond the ordinary screen of consciousness, called the subconscious mind. It is this subconscious area of mind where mind-body interactions appear most prevalent. It is within this jurisdiction of the mind that the primary area of exploration was conducted in this study. This work is empirical and quantitative in nature; it is not necessary to accept the notion of a subconscious mind to accept the results. However, it is the most parsimonious explanation or framework to contextualize this research, even if the separation of the mind and brain is not accepted. Otherwise the reader may have difficulty integrating all of the data points presented.

It is beyond the scope of this research to theorize beyond a simple operational definition of beliefs and subconscious beliefs. For the purposes of this study, repetitive thoughts were considered beliefs. Subconscious beliefs were defined as beliefs that occur beyond ordinary conscious awareness or attention.

Specific Research Questions and Hypothesis

The purpose of this research study and inquiry was to examine and attempt to answer the research question: Does altering subconscious beliefs remove limitations on human capability?

Specifically, the primary research question is: Does removing the subconscious belief in an object of visual obstruction remove the limitations on vision created by the object of visual obstruction? The secondary research question is: Does removing the subconscious belief in limitations on vision remove the limitations on vision? The primary hypothesis states that removing the subconscious belief in an object of visual obstruction will remove the limitations on vision. If the primary hypothesis is supported, the research question would point to the possibility of nonphysical sight. The secondary hypothesis states that creating a subconscious belief in visual improvement will result in improved vision.

Personal Significance

The idea for this research originated in a story told by Talbot (1991) in his book *The Holographic Universe*. Talbot shared an event at a dinner party that he attended where a stage hypnotist was present. The hypnotist stood behind a person sitting at the dinner table and had given a posthypnotic suggestion to another person sitting at the table that the person he was standing behind would be invisible to them. According to Talbot, the person hypnotized was able to guess the object that was held in the hypnotist's hand that was behind the person the hypnotist was standing behind.

As a hypnotist, this was intriguing to the author. A negative hallucination, as just described, is the sixth and deepest level on the Arons hypnotic depth scale used by the National Guild of Hypnotists (Harte, 1991), which will be described in greater detail in the research method section. In 2010, a relative was visiting who was not aware that this writer was a hypnotist. At this person's request, nontherapeutic hypnosis was performed. At one point, an amnesia-induced posthypnotic suggestion was given that created a negative hallucination. In this case a large living room couch was rendered invisible. This person was able to guess correctly how many fingers were held out behind the invisible couch a few times, before beginning to guess incorrectly when an observer walked over in disbelief. It was this event that was the precursor to this research.

On a more personal note, in 2002 or 2003 this writer suffered from temporary blindness in the left eye. The hemorrhage of a blood vessel in the left eye created a black mass covering the whole field of vision. The physician was planning to remove the vitreous of the eye, which is the jellylike substance that makes up the bulk of the eye and gives it its shape. It was through what can only be described as deep self-hypnosis and affirmative prayer that the mass of blood obscuring vision was absorbed, restoring vision in the eye without the need of surgery. This personal experience strengthened the author's commitment to the healing potential and value of hypnotherapy.

Purpose, Significance, and Importance of the Study

As will be seen in the research method section to follow, this research study was deliberately bold and direct. This approach was taken to apply the scientific method clearly and concisely to the research questions. The current study sought to utilize hypnotic depth and susceptibility and test the limits of the effect of altering subconscious beliefs on human capability. The following research was necessary because it may enhance self-awareness for humans and facilitate a greater understanding of their role in the physical universe.

We do not know the limits to human capabilities and the influence of conscious beliefs and subconscious beliefs on human capabilities. Parapsychological research has been at the cutting edge of exploration in this arena. This research investigated and tested the limits of subconscious beliefs and human capability by exploring the effect of altering subconscious beliefs on visual capabilities.

Study Design

This primary research used a quantitative, single study design. Participants were treated with three conditions measuring vision. Vision was measured prior to hypnosis, after a posthypnotic suggestion was given to improve vision, and one final time after an amnesia-induced posthypnotic suggestion was given creating a negative hallucination (rendering an object invisible) regarding an object of visual obstruction that was placed in front of the eye chart. The total number of participants was measured for visual improvement. A subset of individuals able to achieve the negative hallucination was measured for visual accuracy.

Organization of the Study

The following literature review focuses on hypnosis mind-body healing or interaction, viewed within the context of human potentiality resulting from altering subconscious beliefs via hypnosis. Expanding on the theme of human potentiality, parapsychological studies involving hypnosis are reviewed. This is followed by the research method, results, and discussion of the study.

Chapter 2: Literature Review

The purpose of this chapter is to explore and present a wide range of studies where hypnosis has been utilized to create a mind-body effect. After examining the area of hypnosis, mind-body phenomena and exploration of psi, or as often called, parapsychological studies, will be conducted. The uniqueness of this study and its rationale will then be presented.

Hypnosis and Mind-body Healing

In reviewing the literature available on hypnosis mind-body phenomena, it seems logical to begin in the area of pain and pain management, as this is a widely accepted area in which hypnosis has been applied. According to Spiegel (2013), in the mid 1800s British surgeon James Esdaile was operating in India. Esdaile was successfully employing hypnosis for improving surgical outcomes. Hypnosis was also used for pain management and as a general anesthesia. These were reportedly often major surgeries that included amputations (Spiegel, 2013). Esdaile (1846) detailed the laborious process of what was then known as mesmerism. In addition to suggestion, this included mesmeric passes that were literally passing of the hands over the body without physical contact that lasted hours. Esdaile's cases were serious and his results positive regarding reduced infections, pain, and success of surgical outcomes.

Hypnosis and pain. More recent research conducted during invasive renal and vascular surgery supported the observation that self-hypnosis during and after surgery reduced pain and anxiety and stabilized blood pressure (Lang et al., 2000). Hypnosis as a pain management technique has also been shown to be effective with acute and chronic pain (Patterson & Jensen, 2003). A meta-analysis supported a potentially broad application for hypnosis regarding pain management (Montgomery, DuHamel, & Redd, 2000). Another meta-analysis supported hypnosis as an effective approach for a broad application of pain management for chronic pain.

In many of the studies reviewed, hypnosis often outperformed psychoeducation, attention, and physical therapy (Elkins, Jensen, & Patterson, 2007). A greater sense of well-being and reduced stress often accompanied hypnotic pain reduction (Jensen et al., 2006).

Liossi and Hatira (1999) have suggested that hypnosis may be an effective pain management approach for those receiving cancer treatment. Hypnosis appeared more effective than cognitive behavioral therapy when dealing with procedural-related pain, particularly in the area of behavioral stress and anxiety (Liossi & Hatira, 1999). A study of pediatric cancer patients aged 6 to 16 who were receiving regular lumbar punctures as part of the cancer treatment found patients reporting less behavioral distress, anxiety, and pain through the use of hypnosis. Reportedly the effect diminished slightly when patients were transitioned from receiving hypnosis to continuing with self-hypnosis (Liossi & Hatira, 2003).

Another study involving pediatric cancer patients receiving a lumbar puncture showed that hypnosis was more effective when combined with an analgesic cream than the analgesic cream alone. A correlation between those with greater susceptibility to hypnotic suggestion and increased effect was also seen. Those with a higher level of hypnotic suggestibility benefited from the increased effect when hypnosis was used on its own without the analgesic cream (Liossi, White, & Hatira, 2006).

It is worthwhile to note that hypnosis appears to be an effective treatment for pain, although the ancillary mental health benefits when dealing with physical pain should not be disregarded. Several controlled studies of cancer patients evaluated by meta-analysis revealed that hypnosis was an effective approach to reducing the nausea and vomiting often associated with chemotherapy (Richardson et al., 2007). Terminally ill cancer patients not only had less anxiety and depression, but they also achieved a higher quality of life (Liossi & White, 2001).

Hypnosis pain reduction associated with cancer and its treatment is not limited to children. For instance, adult bone marrow transplant recipients experienced less pain with hypnosis (Syrjala, Cummings, & Donaldson, 1992). In one case study, a woman unable to receive anesthesia had a tumor removed on her thigh. The only anesthetic used was hypnosis. The woman's blood pressure or heart rate did not rise during the surgery (Facco, Pasquali, Zanette, & Casiglia, 2013). A larger study of 20 women undergoing breast biopsies with brief hypnosis prior to surgery resulted in less pain and anxiety after the procedure (Montgomery, Weltz, Seltz, & Bovbjerg, 2002). Void of negative side effects, hypnosis, and particularly self-hypnosis, appears effective in high stress situations, including surgery, at reducing anxiety (Hammond, 2010).

A case study of a patient with multiple sclerosis demonstrated that 2 weeks of hypnotic imagery and posthypnotic suggestions alleviated the symptom of double vision, and the patient regained the ability to walk and reported less pain without the use of drugs (Dane, 1996). More recently, Jensen et al. (2009) demonstrated success with multiple sclerosis in larger studies. Patients taught self-hypnosis for pain reduction faired better than those undergoing progressive muscle relaxation (Jensen et al., 2009).

Hypnosis in the form of *virtual reality hypnosis* using a computer screen appeared effective at reducing pain for those experiencing traumatic injuries. Subjective measures of pain 8 hours after treatment produced better results as an adjunct to standard care compared to standard care alone (Patterson, Jensen, Wiechman, & Sharar, 2010). Virtual reality hypnosis was successful in reducing pain resulting from multiple fractures (Teeley et al., 2012). Compared to a control group, those receiving hypnosis in an intensive care unit, suffering from burn wounds, saw increased opioid effectiveness, reduced pain and anxiety, as well as a reduction in the need for anesthesia and a reduction in skin grafting (Berger et al., 2010). Plastic surgery patients also experienced less pain and anxiety, as well as less vomiting and nausea and an increased sense of satisfaction (Roediger, Joris, & Lenny, 1995). In addition to reducing need for medication, hypnosis has been demonstrated to reduce pain and anxiety, and increase stability regarding vital signs, for those receiving plastic surgery (Faymonville et al., 1997).

The above studies demonstrate that hypnosis is a versatile treatment for pain resulting from a variety of causes. Hypnosis also appears as a potent adjunct to other pain management treatments, and may reduce the side effects or even enhance the effects of other treatments. This application of hypnosis should not be understated. It seems that hypnosis may be an untapped resource and has a potentially broad role in the area of pain management.

Hypnosis mental health benefits. Several studies using hypnosis to anchor a sense of security and control with pleasant smells appeared effective in dealing with combat posttraumatic stress, panic disorder, and phobias (Abramowitz & Lichtenberg, 2009). Hypnosis used in conjunction with antidepressants saw greater results than antidepressants alone for the treatment of combat-related posttraumatic stress syndrome (Abramowitz, Barak, Ben-Avi, & Knobler, 2008). Hypnosis combined with cognitive behavioral therapy was effective at treating posttraumatic stress disorder (PTSD), and after a 6-month follow-up had the least number of people re-experiencing PTSD symptoms when compared to a control group and a group receiving only cognitive behavioral therapy (Bryant, Moulds, Guthrie, & Nixon, 2005).

A 12-week hypnosis study exploring occupational and work stress using hypnosis recordings resulted in better eating habits, less perfectionism, and less negative self-talk and criticism. Moreover, hypnosis was also associated with physiological changes. Ensuing blood tests demonstrated a lower level of an inflammatory cytokine linked with stress, called IL-6

(Schoen & Nowack, 2013). Other research showed hypnosis effective at reducing stress and increasing a sense of well-being, showing a relationship of hypnotic suggestibility with reduced stress and increased well-being. A moderate hypnotic suggestibility level revealed a positive benefit, although the effect was greater with those who achieved greater hypnotic suggestibility (Cardeña, Svensson, & Hejdström, 2013). Stress, anxiety, and procrastination were all reduced in a study using hypnosis to treat generalized anxiety disorder (Craciun, Holdevici, & Craciun, 2012). Further research indicated that the intensity of stressful memories and events were reduced by hypnosis, timeline therapy, and neurolinguistic programming (Ahmad & Zaman, 2011).

According to Yapko (2010a), despite the fact that many therapists are not trained in hypnosis and are often unaware of its efficacy, hypnosis is an effective method for the treatment of depression. Therapists can incorporate well-established protocols into a hypnosis session (Yapko, 1993). Hypnosis also reduces cognitive inflexibility and facilitates the learning of new thought patterns and reducing repetitive thinking associated with depression (Yapko, 2010b). A controlled study compared cognitive behavioral therapy alone and hypnosis combined with cognitive behavioral therapy, with the result that the group that also received hypnosis faired significantly better (Alladin & Alibhai, 2007). Yexley (2007) found that hypnosis may also reduce postpartum depression.

A case study showed hypnosis to be effective in treating a severe driving phobia resulting from an accident. After 16 sessions the participant reported a full recovery and was driving without anxiety (T. Kraft & D. Kraft, 2004). In another case study, a combination of hypnosis, solution-focused therapy, and psychodynamics was successful in treating panic disorder and agoraphobia (D. Kraft, 2012). Another case history demonstrated the success of hypnosis in treating a panic disorder and phobia of flying (Volpe & Nash, 2012). Of those suffering from claustrophobia interfering with the ability to have an MRI, 90% saw a successful result after hypnosis (Velloso, Duprat, Martins, & Scoppetta, 2010). In a dental case involving a blood phobia with a gagging reflux, hypnosis was successful in removing the gagging reflux and the blood phobia was relieved, allowing teeth to be removed (Noble, 2002). Although there are limitations to the value of individual case studies for demonstrating clear efficacy, such cases do point to the value of conducting larger studies. The several meta-analyses cited here are more valuable in building confidence in hypnosis as an evidence-based treatment modality.

A meta-analysis of hypnosis combined with cognitive behavioral therapy in the area of weight loss showed that those receiving hypnosis fared better than 70% of those who did not, and also saw long-term benefits (Kirsch, Montgomery, & Sapirstein, 1995). In a controlled study regarding smoking cessation, hypnosis outperformed behavioral therapy (Carmody et al., 2008). Another study on smoking, using only three hypnosis sessions, had 81% of participants discontinue smoking, and a 48% retention rate after a year (Elkins & Rajab, 2004). Another hypnosis smoking study using carbon monoxide testing revealed 40% were not smoking after 26 weeks (Elkins, Marcus, Bates, Hasan Rajab, & Cook, 2006).

Treatment of substance addiction has shown some success with hypnosis. In a controlled study at a methadone clinic, after 6 months 94% of participants who were able to stop taking methadone were abstinent of any drug use (Manganiello, 1984). A hypnosis study involving heroin addicts receiving group hypnosis once a week were 100% heroin free after 6 months (Kaminsky, Rosca, Budowski, Korin, & Yakhnich, 2007). Another study of substance abuse with participants receiving daily hypnosis sessions for 20 days resulted in 77% abstinence after a year (Potter, 2004).

Guided imagery was used in a controlled study with participants who had reconstructive knee surgery over the course of 10 sessions, showing increased knee strength and reduced pain and anxiety (Cupal & Brewer, 2001). The term guided imagery, which is a subset or technique of hypnosis, is sometimes used by practitioners to avoid dealing with negative connotations associated with hypnosis. It should be noted that there is some evidence that using the term hypnosis actually increases the effects of suggestions (Schoenberger, Kirsch, Gearan, Montgomery, & Pastyrnak, 1998). The possible underlying fear or stigma associated with hypnosis may enhance its increased effectiveness. In a brief four-session treatment, hypnosis along with psychological education greatly reduced chronic low back pain (Tan, Fukui, Jensen, Thornby, & Waldman, 2009).

In the area of mental health hypnosis may be a useful approach to a variety of issues. Again, hypnosis appears to be effective on its own, yet it also seems an effective host to other therapeutic approaches. One conclusion that may be drawn from the research cited is that hypnosis may enhance other therapeutic treatments and also accelerate the effect of various treatments.

Hypnosis, headaches, and tinnitus. The body of research presented in this literature review echoes a well-known fact among clinicians, which is that there are no known serious side effects to hypnosis itself. Rare, minor adverse reactions include headache, drowsiness, dizziness, anxiety, or distress (Harte, 1991). Migraine headaches are another area of pain management where hypnosis seems effective with no adverse effects. Such treatment meets the clinical psychology guidelines as a well-established treatment (Hammond, 2007). A review of outpatient records between 1988 and 2001 showed self-hypnosis effective in reducing the frequency and intensity of headaches (Kohen & Zajac, 2007). Tinnitus, which is a consistent or persistent ringing or noise in the ears or head, has no known cure. Hypnosis has been shown to produce immediate and lasting effects in the treatment of debilitating tinnitus (Gajan et al., 2011). While other treatments such as masking and attentiveness did not yield any results, self-hypnosis significantly reduced the severity of tinnitus (Attias et al., 1993).

Hypnosis and sleep. The following hypnosis studies are fascinating because they not only show the efficacy of hypnosis with improving sleep, which has broad health benefits, but they also show changes in the brain. These brain changes demonstrate physiological changes as a direct result of hypnotic suggestion.

Hypnosis is effective at treating the insomnia, anxiety, and depression that result from tinnitus (Mirzamani, Bahrami, Moghtaderi, & Namegh, 2012). After completing a 28-day inpatient treatment for tinnitus, 90.5% of those with subacute tinnitus and 88.3% with chronic tinnitus had a decrease in severity and the effect was stable after 3- and 6-month follow-ups (Ross, Lange, Unterrainer, & Laszig, 2007).

In a controlled study, hypnosis has been demonstrated to improve slow wave pattern sleep by 80%. Slow wave pattern sleep increases cellular repair and a healthy immune system. Researchers asserted that the slow wave pattern sleep resulted specifically from the suggestion to sleep deeply, not merely expectations for deep sleep (Cordi, Schlarb, & Rasch, 2014). Further research supports that hypnosis is successful with treating insomnia. A case study of a girl with type 1 diabetes saw positive results utilizing hypnosis (Perfect & Elkins, 2010). Self-hypnosis taught over one or two sessions has been effective with treating children suffering from insomnia (Hawkins & Polemikos, 2002). Other research with children suffering from insomnia showed that 90% of those struggling to fall asleep improved, and 87% eliminated the problem of waking up as the result of aches and pains (Anbar & Slothower, 2006). Hypnosis may be effective in increasing deep sleep in the elderly by as much as 57% and may increase cognitive function. Slow wave pattern sleep was increased, as well as prefrontal cognitive patterns (Cordi, Hirsiger, Mérillat, & Rasch, 2015). Further research on a younger population supported that hypnotic suggestion increased slow wave pattern sleep and may be effective at treating sleep disturbances (Cordi, Rossier, & Rasch, 2018).

The physiological changes resulting from hypnosis and hypnotic suggestion in these studies may be considered a parapsychological effect. The altering of subconscious beliefs via hypnotic suggestion created changes in brain function. If a certain degree of dualism exists between mind and body, in a sense mind-body interaction of this sort may be parapsychological.

Hypnosis, arthritis, sickle cell anemia, and Parkinson's. Rheumatoid arthritis, which includes an underlying autoimmune reaction as well as joint pain, stiffness, and swelling, was treated with hypnosis. A controlled study with a relaxation group and a hypnosis group utilized individualized imagery. The hypnosis group showed positive results in subjective measures such as joint function and an objective measure in the form of a blood test showing a reduction in the autoimmune reaction. At follow-up for participants who practiced hypnotic imagery regularly, both measures were more significant (Horton-Hausknecht, Mitzdorf, & Melchart, 2000).

A small case study involving several pediatric participants with sickle cell anemia showed that hypnosis reduced frequency and intensity of pain episodes (Zeltzer, Dash, & Holland, 1979). A larger study with sickle cell anemia participants conducted over 18 months combining cognitive behavioral therapy with hypnosis showed a significant reduction in pain. This led researchers to conclude that most mild and moderate pain episodes were eliminated, leaving only severe pain episodes (Dinges et al., 1997).

A case study with a patient with Parkinson's disease showed promising results using hypnosis and self-hypnosis to reduce tremors (Wain, Amen, & Jabbari, 1990). In another case study, researchers reported that according to sensors, a Parkinson's patient had a 94% reduction in tremors after three weekly hypnosis sessions. The patient also reported less pain, anxiety, and depression. Also reported were an improved quality of life, libido, and sleep (Elkins, Sliwinski, Bowers, & Encarnacion, 2013). In a larger controlled study using relaxation and guided imagery, all 20 participants had a dramatic reduction in tremors (Schlesinger, Benyakov, Erikh, Suraiya, & Schiller, 2009).

The physiological changes in these studies are significant because they again show a direct mind-body interaction through hypnotic suggestion. These changes appear in function such as the reduction of tremors. The changes also were evident in blood tests. The altering of subconscious beliefs through hypnosis created a functional and systemic physiological change.

Hypnosis and changes in the brain. Hypnosis may also be effective in treating phantom limb pain; a small study using positron emission topography (PET) scans showed resulting activity in the area of the brain associated with motor and sensory processing (Rosén, Willoch, Bartenstein, Berner, & Røsjø, 2001). A study with fibromyalgia patients also using positron emission topography (PET) scans showed that hypnosis-induced analgesia is a dynamic process involving multiple regions of the brain. PET scans demonstrated that hypnosis-induced analgesia involved both cortical and subcortical regions of the brain (Wik, Fischer, Bragée, Finer, & Fredrikson, 1999).

Another study with fibromyalgia patients using functional magnetic resonance imaging (fMRI) explored the effect of simple pain reduction suggestions versus pain reduction suggestions given to hypnotized participants. The fMRI showed changes to the brain with either condition receiving the suggestion; however, the group that was hypnotized while given these pain reduction suggestions showed an amplified effect on the fMRI (Derbyshire, Whalley, & Oakley, 2009). Cognitive behavioral therapy combined with hypnosis outperformed drugs and cognitive therapy alone in treating pain associated with fibromyalgia (Castel, Salvat, Sala, & Rull, 2009). Analgesia suggestions for patients while hypnotized were more effective than pain reduction and relaxation suggestions while relaxed (Castel, Pérez, Sala, Padrol, & Rull, 2007).

Brain changes occurring due to hypnosis and hypnotic suggestion are a fascinating example of a direct mind-body reaction. Research using fMRI data further demonstrated the hypnosis mind-body interaction as well as the potential for further research with hypnosis using advanced technology. Hypnotic suggestion given to create pain potentially highlighted the neural pathway for the immediate creation of pain (Derbyshire, Whalley, Stenger, & Oakley, 2004). A reported case of an apparent allergic reaction due to a hypnotic suggestion may demonstrate a more pronounced example of thoughts influencing the physical body. In this scenario, the psychologist was not aware that a dental patient was allergic to Novocain and when the hypnotic suggestion to achieve a Novocain-like numbness was given, the patient had an allergic reaction involving a swollen cheek. Once the cause was realized, hypnotic suggestions to countermand the effect were given (Guttman & Ball, 2013).

The changes in the brain and brain patterns of activity measured in the above referenced studies are empirical. These studies used state-of-the-art contemporary methods to measure brain function. The altering of subconscious beliefs via hypnotic suggestion has created actual changes to the brain and body. This is a direct mind-body interaction involving the brain itself.

Hypnosis and childbirth. The mind-body effect of hypnosis is also evident in the area of childbirth. Hypnosis may be effective at prolonging pregnancy and in some cases actually stopping preterm labor (Corey Brown & Corydon Hammond, 2007). One study, which measured a control group and a group using self-hypnosis, resulted in 53% of the control group needing epidurals and only 36% of the self-hypnosis group needing epidurals and requiring less augmentation (Cyna, Andrew, & McAuliffe, 2006). Those with no prior hypnosis training who were hypnotized during labor received less medication and reported less pain, adding only 45 minutes to labor (Rock, Shipley, & Campbell, 1969). Childbirth involving hypnosis resulted in higher Apgar scores and shorter stage 1 labor (Harmon, Hynan, & Tyre, 1990). Those receiving hypnosis in the first and second trimester also had improved outcomes and fewer complications (Mehl-Madrona, 2004). Hypnosis regarding in vitro fertilization during the actual embryo transfer produced a 76% increase in pregnancy compared to a control group (Levitas et al., 2006). With fewer side effects, hypnosis is as effective as diazepam regarding pregnancy ratio and relaxation (Catoire et al., 2013). A pilot study of women going through menopause utilizing hypnosis resulted in 72% reduction of hot flashes and a 76% reduction in intensity (Elkins, Johnson, Fisher, Sliwinski, & Keith, 2013).

The ability of hypnosis to reduce pain and the need for medications is in itself a very important function. Improved birth outcomes are demonstrating something else. This may be an example of the altering of subconscious beliefs to enhance human capability. Essentially, Apgar scores are a form of early IQ test.

Hypnosis and stroke recovery. One case study with hypnosis and a stroke victim after 5 weeks resulted in the participant regaining partial control of facial muscles and full movement of his arm and leg (Manganiello, 1986). Another study of six chronic stroke victims utilizing hypnosis resulted in increased motor function and grip strength as well as range of motion requiring less effort. Hypnotherapy also produced increased motivation and self-awareness as well as a more positive outlook (Diamond, Davis, Schaechter, & Howe, 2006). A randomized pilot study of stroke victims compared a group using occupational therapy and a group receiving occupational therapy and guided imagery. The group receiving the guided imagery in addition to the occupational therapy improved while the occupational therapy group remained the same (Page, Levine, Sisto, & Johnston, 2001).

According to Siegel (1998), visualizing something and actually doing something is not distinguished in the brain. This claim appears to be supported by research utilizing a fMRI as visualizing something and actually seeing it use similar parts of the brain (Ganis, Thompson, & Kosslyn, 2004). Mental imagery produces a similar autonomic response and blood flow in the brain as occurs when doing the actual activity (Decety, 1996). Doidge (2007) reported that the brain has the ability to restructure itself even among those with disabilities and medical conditions. This brain plasticity or neuroplasticity results from changing thoughts or actions (Doidge, 2007). Other research with using fMRI demonstrated that hypnosis rehabilitated patients with brain damage and improved motor skills. Motor imagery while hypnotized facilitated rehabilitation even in instances where the ability to imagine movements was impaired (Müller, Bacht, Schramm, & Seitz, 2012).

The application of hypnosis and altering subconscious beliefs to enhance the rehabilitation of stroke victims is in itself a phenomenal argument supporting thoughts as directing the body. It may be lost at first glance, because it is a repairing of functions that were lost or damaged, that this is again an issue of human capability being enhanced by hypnosis.

Hypnosis and surgery. Hypnosis in postsurgical situations has been shown to reduce pain and also stabilize blood flow and circulation (Lang et al., 2000). Prior to surgery, hypnosis-guided imagery resulted in fewer complications and hospitalizations, as well as reduced blood loss for patients receiving head and neck surgery (Rapkin, Straubing, & Holroyd, 1991). Another controlled study involving angioplasty surgery noted that the group who received hypnosis before and during surgery produced higher norepinephrine levels, had a reduced need for narcotics necessary for surgery, and also benefited by a 25% increase in the amount of time the balloon at the tip of the catheter was able to be inflated in the arteries (Weinstein & Au, 1991). Those receiving cataract surgery required less intravenous drugs, reported higher quality experience, and demonstrated greater cognitive function at discharge (Flore, 2014).

Hypnosis and regeneration. Research at Massachusetts General Hospital, which included an examination of radiological data as well as orthopedic assessment for patients with bone fractures, showed that the hypnosis group faired noticeably better than the control group. Bone fracture edge healing was noticeably improved for hypnosis patients, and hypnosis patients also had reduced pain, increased mobility, and less pain-killer drug use (Ginandes & Rosenthal, 1999). In a study where medical staff blinded to the study evaluated mammoplasty patients' incision wounds, those receiving hypnosis saw accelerated healing (Ginandes, Brooks, Sando, Jones, & Aker, 2003). In another clinical pilot study demonstrating anatomical changes as a result of hypnosis, the cartilage between finger joints, or the metacarpus, was elongated during rapid hypnotic finger induction (Eitner, 2006).

Some research has suggested that hypnosis is effective with burn wound healing. Blinded medical staff evaluated patients selected with symmetrical burn wounds who were given hypnotic suggestions to accelerate healing only on one side of the body and verified the results, which conformed to the suggestions. One patient healed equally on both sides of the body; however, the other four patients healed on one side of the body as suggested (Moore & Kaplan,

1983). A meta-analysis showed hypnosis patients with better surgical outcomes than 89% of control patients (Montgomery, David, Winkel, Silverstein, & Bovbjerg, 2002).

These studies again are supporting a position that hypnosis and hypnotic suggestion altering subconscious beliefs creates a mind-body interaction. In the case of bone fracture regeneration, the effect moved beyond soft tissue to bone. This may help to question where and how the limits and effect of altering subconscious beliefs should be placed.

Hypnosis and blood flow. Hypertension, or high blood pressure, has also been treated successfully and eliminated with hypnosis in a controlled study (Deabler, Fidel, Dillenkoffer, & Elder, 1973). In a study of hemophiliacs, the group who used self-hypnosis had a significant reduction in the need for clotting factor concentrate (Swirsky-Sacchetti & Margolis, 1986). A case study with a patient with hemophilia undergoing a dental procedure, who would normally need a transfusion during the procedure, received hypnosis in addition to anesthesia and medications. The patient did not require a transfusion and did not bleed during the procedure (Dubin & Shapiro, 1974).

In a study with hypnosis and Raynaud's disease in participants of varying ages, skin temperature rose during hypnosis 1.4 degrees Celsius and to 2.7 degrees Celsius after hypnotic suggestion. There was a 63% increase in capillary blood flow. Some of the participants also had improvements with complications involving diabetes due to blood circulation (Grabowska, 1971). A case study with a highly hypnotizable participant with Raynaud's disease showed a fourfold increase in blood supply (Conn & Mott, Jr., 1984).

Hypnosis, diabetes, alopecia, and skin disorders. There is limited research with hypnosis and diabetes. One study tested participants who were hypnotized to recall the worst life memory. Their glucose levels were regularly tested against a control period and resulted in drops in glucose levels (Vandenbergh, Sussman, & Titus, 1966). Healthy people hypnotized to imagine eating food saw an increase in insulin production in their blood without a change in glucose levels (Goldfine, Abraira, Gruenewald, & Goldstein, 1970). Hypnosis may be an effective adjunct for those with diabetes for stabilizing glucose levels and addressing complications such as peripheral vascular issues (Xu & Cardeña, 2007).

Another autoimmune disease called alopecia, which results in the loss of body hair, showed promising results after only three to eight hypnosis sessions. Used either alone or as an adjunct to other treatments, 12 of 28 participants had positive results with hypnosis, including some with severe cases that included loss of eyebrow hair (Willemsen, Vanderlinden, Deconinck, & Roseeuw, 2006).

Hypnosis has been shown effective at treating certain skin diseases. One case study showed a full remission from an incurable and rare disease that produces hard, dry-like scales on the skin, called ichthyosis (Mason, 1952). A controlled study showed highly susceptible hypnotic participants seeing significant improvements in psoriasis (Tausk & Whitmore, 1999). Hypnosis also reduced the severity of skin surface damage with eczema (Sokel, Christie, Kent, & Lansdown, 1993), and produced very positive results with warts (Noll, 1994).

Hypnosis, asthma, and allergies. Hypnosis can reduce symptoms from skin responses with participants with asthma and hay fever (Fry, Mason, & Pearson, 1964). Other research with allergies resulted in 76% of those taught self-hypnosis reporting improvements in symptoms and a reduction in medications (Madrid, Rostel, Pennington, & Murphy, 1995). Using a histamine skin-prick test and highly hypnotizable participants, a controlled study showed hypnosis reducing allergic reactions. Hypnotic suggestion also demonstrated the ability to increase reaction time in one arm and reduce it in the other (Zachariae, Bjerring, & Arendt-Nielsen, 1989). Hypnosis has also prevented allergic skin reactions to poison ivy (Barber, 1978).

Other research on asthma showed a hypnosis group producing better results than a group receiving antispasmodics. The hypnosis group improved on wheezing and used less medication. Those who reached deeper hypnotic states and used self-hypnosis had the best outcomes (Maher-Loughnan, Macdonald, Mason, & Fry, 1962). Other research produced similar results regarding participants who were hypnotized and also practiced self-hypnosis (Maher-Loughnan, 1970).

Another asthma study also saw participants who were able to reach deeper states of hypnosis as showing improved results (Collison, 1975). Other research resulted in participants achieving a 50% improvement based on pulmonary function (Aronoff, Aronoff, & Peck, 1975). Those with asthma who underwent hypnosis did better than a control group when pulmonary function was measured after running on a treadmill (Ben-Zvi, Spohn, Young, & Kattan, 1982).

Hypnosis and bowel disorders. After hypnotherapy 76% of those with irritable bowel disease reported an improved quality of life, 60% stopped taking corticosteroids, and 26% reported total remission (Miller & Whorwell, 2008). Irritable bowel syndrome also responded well to hypnosis with long-lasting effects and a reduction in medication use over time (Gonsalkorale & Whorwell, 2005). Functional dyspepsia also had very positive results with hypnosis, seeing long-term effects and dramatic reduction of medication use (Calvert, Houghton, Cooper, Morris, & Whorwell, 2002).

Hypnosis and immune system enhancement. Hypnosis may have an effect on immune system function. In addition to increasing a sense of well-being, breast cancer patients who were treated with hypnosis-induced guided imagery saw an increase in natural killer cells (NK cells). NK cells attack tumor formation. However, the effect wore off once the treatment stopped

(Bakke, Purtzer, & Newton, 2002). Other research on women with advanced breast cancer showed relaxation and guided imagery increasing NK cells as well as T-cells and Lak cells (Eremin et al., 2009).

Participants diagnosed with cancer, AIDS, viral infections, and other medical conditions were treated with a 30-minute audiotape including relaxation suggestions and guided imagery over a 90-day period. Participants did not receive any other treatment. After 90 days, there was a significant increase in white blood cell count (Donaldson, 2000). A hypnosis study with healthy participants given posthypnotic suggestions to reduce stress, along with balancing the immune system and neuroendocrine system, resulted in an altered T-cell response after just three sessions (Wood et al., 2003).

Hypnosis and performance. In the area of performance enhancement there are a few case studies showing hypnosis as effective with sports performance. A small hypnosis study with five basketball participants resulted in an improvement in mean 3-point scores for all participants (Pates, Cummings, & Maynard, 2002). Another small study with five participants using hypnosis resulted in all participants increasing their mean golf putting scores (Pates, Oliver, & Maynard, 2001). A single-subject design on a European pro golfer also produced positive results, with the golfer improving his mean stroke average (Pates, 2013). A case study showed hypnosis improving archery over a 20-week period (Robazza & Bortoli, 1995). Another case study showed positive results for a gymnast (Newmark, 2012).

Research has reported group hypnosis for improved test scores on college achievement tests when compared to control groups (Schreiber, 1997). Some evidence indicates that posthypnotic suggestion may improve test scores (Hammer, 1954). Procedural learning, which relies on implicit memories, may be enhanced with hypnosis (Nemeth, Janacsek, Polner, &

Kovacs, 2013). Compared to controls, self-hypnosis may be effective at increasing reading comprehension and vocabulary (Fillmer, 1980). Posthypnotic suggestion also improved reading compared to controls, especially for more susceptible participants (Koe & Oldridge, 1988). Creativity may also be enhanced with hypnosis in real-world situations (Sanders, 1976). Another study used the Torrance Test of creativity and the hypnosis group faired significantly better than controls (Gur & Reyher, 1976). Other research with artists struggling with creative blocks in various fields showed positive results with the hypnosis group (Barrios & Singer, 1981).

Hypnosis and vision. Research has supported the possibility that hypnosis may affect eyesight. Braid (1843) reported cases of patients having improved vision after hypnosis. There is a published case study reporting that vision spontaneously improved during the hypnosis session, then returned to normal afterward (Davison & Singleton, 1967). As will be mentioned later, the lasting effects of visual improvement with hypnosis are still unclear. In cases of people suffering from multiple personality disorder there have been documented changes in vision for different alters (Miller, 1989). There was also a social psychology experiment utilizing the power of suggestion involving a flight simulator. The study demonstrated improved vision for participants taking on the role of pilots when compared to the control group (Langer, Djikic, Pirson, Madenci, & Donohue, 2010). One study demonstrated that participants who were hypnotized not only saw improved vision while hypnotized, but also were given posthypnotic suggestions that resulted in improved vision afterward. Those who had the worst vision saw the greatest improvement (Graham & Leibowitz, 1972). Using tape-recorded hypnotic suggestions may improve visual acuity (Sheehan, Smith, & Forrest, 1982). Other research showed improved vision after hypnotic suggestion (Kay, 1992). These and other findings have been critiqued as not representing hypnosis as an effective long-term technique to deal with myopia, and assert that hypnosis may increase memorization, cognitive functions, and perceptual learning (Raz, Zephrani, Schweizer, & Marinoff, 2004).

The studies cited thus far in this literature review cover a wide array of conditions for which hypnosis and hypnotic suggestion have been effective. The altering of subconscious beliefs in the hypnotic condition to produce physiological changes appears consistent across a wide range of physical issues. These results are dealing with the regeneration of lost abilities or restoring normal functioning, the exception being reducing or eliminating pain, which could be viewed as an enhanced ability.

One important conclusion can be drawn from the body of research studies cited. This is that the altering of subconscious beliefs appears to influence what are generally considered autonomic processes. The regeneration of bone, manipulation of blood flow, wound healing, autoimmune and allergic responses are conventionally considered decoupled from thought and beyond the reach of intentions and thought. It may very well be that these capabilities and functions are beyond conscious thoughts and beliefs. It is reasonable, however, at this point to consider not only if these capabilities are influenced by subconscious beliefs, but to what degree they fall under such influence.

The area of hypnotic suggestion and visual improvement is one area that this study re-explored briefly as a secondary measure. Improving vision in those who are nearsighted would fall within the parameters of the studies cited above in that it would be dealing with restoring lost or impaired functioning. In cases of those participating in the study who have normal vision, to begin with an improvement in vision resulting from hypnotic suggestion would infer enhanced capability rather than simply restoring normal functioning. First, a review of parapsychological studies is required as this is an area of inquiry that directly explores human potentiality. The primary focus of this study was to test the limits of hypnosis and human potentiality. Although there is scant research with hypnosis and parapsychological or psi research, that is the first area that will be addressed.

Parapsychological Research

Hypnosis and psi/ESP phenomena. Despite what may be considered a cultural taboo on paranormal investigations among the scientific community, there is continued evidence in support of psychic phenomena (Cardeña, 2014). Since the 1800s, mediumship and supernormal or paranormal ability have been attributed to capacities in the subconscious mind (Esdaile, 1852). This view changed in the late 1800s and early 1900s among many in the scientific community. The paranormal has never been fully accepted by the scientific community and the paranormal as part of the subconscious and dissociation literature has been largely suppressed (Alvarado, 2014).

There appears to be a limited amount of research using hypnosis in the parapsychological literature. In a psychokinetic test on dice throwing and hypnosis, where participants attempted to produce a specific number, the results were statistically significant (Rhine, 1946). Sargent (1978) conducted research using ESP cards, leading the researcher to conclude that hypnosis was a psi-conducive state because the hypnosis group produced significant results compared to the group that was awake during the study. A controlled replication study did demonstrate that hypnosis produced significant psi results while a waking-state group produced chance results on psi testing (Sargent, 1978). At first glance, hypnosis-enhancing psi effects appear to be supported by a meta-analysis of 25 studies (Stanford & Stein, 1994). However, the researchers considered this effect nonconclusive because the significance of hypnosis in these studies was only prevalent when the comparison condition preceded the hypnosis condition and the significance of hypnosis was due to lack of psi in the comparison condition.

In another study, the hypnogogic or hypnotic state itself produced a greater psi effect. Study participants who were hypnotized showed an improved ESP ability. The hypnosis or hypnogogic state outperformed self-relaxation when attempting to determine a target in a separate room (Del Prete & Tressoldi, 2005). Follow-up research was supportive of the ability of the hypnotic state and hypnotic suggestion to enhance ESP (Tressoldi & Del Prete, 2007). Other researchers have concluded that dissociation may mediate effects of hypnotizability and psi effects (Cardeña, Marcusson-Clavertz, & Wasmuth, 2009). More specific inquiry into the issue of whether hypnosis influences psi or ESP was conducted in a pilot study examining the connection between hypnotic susceptibility and an ESP effect. This study resulted in a significant effect with hypnotic susceptibility on ESP tasks. When a group with higher hypnotic susceptibility and lower hypnotic susceptibility were compared, the higher hypnotic susceptibility group showed a greater effect (Parra & Argibay, 2013).

In deep hypnosis some of the perceptual changes that have been reported are body image alterations, distortions of time, sense, perception, and meaning. Awareness, affect, attention, and imagery all appear altered in this state. It may be that distinct states better describe this hypnosis phenomena rather than a continuum of one state (Cardeña, 2005). Deep hypnosis has been reported to simulate many of the characteristics of near-death experiences and out-of-body experiences (Tart, 1970). Recent research in out-of-body experiences (OBEs) induced by hypnosis yielded certain benefits for researchers, in particular the ability to ask the hypnotized participants questions. Of the answers given by the six participants in this study, there was minimal commonality in their answers although there was a commonality among the participants' reports in the existence of at least two distinct nonphysical bodies besides the physical body. These reports correspond to the beliefs in Eastern religious theology such as Vedanta and the Theosophical tradition, which is a combination of Western occultism and Eastern philosophy (Tressoldi et al., 2015).

Neurobiological model for psi. There has been some MRI research with brain-damaged participants and psi. One study involved psychokinesis, or the ability to move objects with the mind. In this study, a random event generator was used in the form of an arrow and its movement to the left or right on a computer screen. Both brain-damaged participants were able to move the arrow to the right and effect sizes were much greater than in normal participants. The researchers concluded that the medial frontal lobes may inhibit psi ability via self-awareness mechanisms, in particular the left medial middle frontal region. Both participants had left frontal lobe damage and the movement was contralateral to the damaged lobes. The researchers also proposed that participants with frontal lobe lesions may be a psi-enriched population to study (Freedman et al., 2018).

This research is interesting within the paranormal area of psi research because it does indirectly support the previously mentioned subconscious and dissociation literature supportive of paranormal effects that originated in the 1800s. Hypnosis, with its effects on dissociation and utilization of the subconscious, may also be supported indirectly with this neurobiological model for psi phenomena. It may be that hypnosis enhances psi effects because it utilizes dissociation and, as a result, enhances psi by simulating the dissociation that occurs with brain-damaged participants, as mentioned above.

Morphic fields and morphic resonance. While his ideas appear largely theoretical in nature, Sheldrake (2012) hypothesized that nature is habitual and proposed the concept of morphic fields and morphic resonance. Morphic fields are probabilistic in nature and resonate with prior versions of morphic fields through a process called morphic resonance. They exist in hierarchies and interact with each other. Morphic fields give rise to and maintain the form of biological systems as well as influence behaviors such as learning and communication, and are a potential explanation for how birds are able to fly and coordinate in a flock as well as schools of fish being able to coordinate when swimming. Hypothesized morphic fields are self-organizing wholes. Vibrational patterns of activity are guided by end points or goals; the most common pathway toward these goals are called creodes (Sheldrake, 2012).

These concepts lend themselves to the support of psi. Sheldrake (2012) also proposed the idea of an extended mind working in a similar fashion as a television set or radio tuning into channels. As such, the brain in this analogy is like the television or radio that needs to be in working order to tune into a channel, yet the actors and musicians do not exist within the television set (Sheldrake, 2012). Braid (1843), who coined the term hypnotism, considered the brain to be an organ of the mind, which is a similar idea.

Correlating morphic fields, archetypes, and subconscious mind. Jung (1936) described archetypes as form without content. This simple notion seems much like a Platonic archetype or eternal idea that guides all form into being. This hypothesis is a top-down approach compared to morphic fields at first glance. Sheldrake (2012) left open the possibility that morphic fields may come into being from top-down processes like Platonic ideas resonating with prior fields, or bottom-up processes more in line with the tradition of Aristotle creating new fields of probability. It may be that within the context of mind-body healing and hypnosis enhancing ESP that the subconscious mind is synonymous with archetypes and morphic fields or is an interface to influence them. The altering of subconscious beliefs, which may be synonymous with attractors or goals within a morphic field, may alter the morphic field itself.

Sheldrake (2012) offered a specific type of morphic field called a perceptual field. In the case of vision, the perceptual field contacts the object being seen (Sheldrake, 2012). This study and the research question, does removing the subconscious belief in an object of visual obstruction remove the limits on vision, may be a test for perceptual fields. R. Sheldrake (personal communication, September 6, 2017) stated that the perceptual field needs to have a direct line of contact with the object being seen; he also asserted that while original and worthwhile, this study is not a good test for perceptual fields because there is not a direct line of contact for the proposed perceptual field and the intended object to be seen via nonphysical sight.

Fields by nature are pliable and in the same way that a magnetic field to a limited degree may go around or through an object, this researcher would argue that a perceptual field should have a degree of pliability and, within reason, could go through or around an object. From an evolutionary perspective this may make sense, as early humans may have benefited from an ability to sense or see through nonphysical means what predators may lurk around a corner.

Research regarding rendering an object invisible and determining if it is possible to see through or around it has never been conducted. If this research is considered within the context of proposed perceptual fields, it would also stand apart from ESP experiments or potentially be viewed as a subset of ESP. If the mechanism of a perceptual field is considered a viable explanation, then this research would still fall within the parameters of ESP since the normal senses are not being utilized; however, the limitations of pliability of a potential perceptual field going through an object or around it would infer limitations of distance around the object or through it that do not appear to apply toward other ESP effects. If support for nonphysical sight is discovered while expanding the human potential, it may be much more bound by time and space than other proposed ESP effects.

Conclusion and Rationale for This Study

Beyond knowing that hypnotic suggestion alters subconscious beliefs, the mechanism underlying hypnosis mind-body healing or hypnosis-enhancing psi effects may never be known. The hypnosis mind-body literature reviewed in this chapter presented a few recurring themes. The hypnosis mind-body effect often appeared enhanced by hypnotic susceptibility and hypnotic depth of the participant. Furthermore, these two factors appear to be related to those who are more susceptible to hypnotic suggestion also being able to achieve deeper states of hypnosis. The hypnosis paranormal research reviewed appears to support that participants who are more susceptible to hypnotic suggestion and those who achieve deeper states of hypnosis appear to have enhanced psi effects. In short, based on the reviewed research, whether it is hypnosis mind-body healing or hypnosis-enhancing psi effects, hypnotic suggestibility and hypnotic depth level appear to enhance effects.

Hypnosis, as already mentioned in the introduction, is an altered state of consciousness where subconscious beliefs may be more easily reconditioned. It appears that, based on the literature reviewed in this study, the altering of subconscious beliefs via hypnosis has created physiological changes in the body. It also appears, based on the paranormal research reviewed, that altering of subconscious beliefs via hypnosis as well as the hypnotic state itself has enhanced ESP. Whether a top-down concept like an archetype is considered, or a potentially top-down and/or bottom-up concept like a morphic field is considered, or even perceptual fields, the mediating factor and the practical mechanism of the subconscious mind and subconscious beliefs may be interchangeable with either descriptive mechanism. In this context, the subconscious mind and subconscious beliefs are called practical because through hypnosis there is an ability to alter them and measure tangible results. It may enrich our research to consider some of the above theories and models that may support this study. Beyond that, it is the practical application of altering subconscious beliefs via hypnosis and the ensuing effect that is of concern to this research study.

Chapter 3: Research Method

The broad general topic that guided this study addressed whether nonphysical sight is possible. To that end, this study addressed the question: Does removing the subconscious belief in an object of visual obstruction remove the limitations on vision created by the object of visual obstruction? Indirectly this question has been addressed in reports of near-death experiences and out-of-body experiences of the blind (Ring & Cooper, 2008). Still, a more quantitative investigation was warranted to determine whether nonphysical sight is possible in a hypnotically induced trance state. The primary hypothesis asserted that by removing the subconscious belief in an object of visual obstruction, the limitations on vision will be removed. If this hypothesis is supported, it can be predicted that participants in this study will be able to see what is on the other side of an object that is obstructing vision.

Secondly, this research asked: Does altering the subconscious belief in visual capability alter vision? The secondary hypothesis asserted that creating a subconscious belief in visual enhancement would result in improved vision. If this hypothesis is supported, it can be predicted that hypnotic suggestion will result in visual improvement. Prior studies on hypnosis and hypnotic suggestion enhancing vision have been criticized to a degree. Critiques attributed visual improvement to attention, memorization, and perceptual learning (Raz et al., 2004). This research sought to address much of this criticism by using a different variation of a standard eye chart when measuring for visual improvement. It did not address concerns of whether such effects on improved vision are temporary and will leave that to potential follow-up research in this area.

Rationale for Selecting Design

This research made use of a *within-subject* design in which participants were treated to three conditions. A control in the form of measuring vision prior to hypnosis was built into the study. The within-subject design was also well suited for this study because the fractionalization (taking a person in and out of hypnosis more than once during one session) is a standard hypnotic deepening technique (Harte, 1991). The deepening of hypnosis was integral to this study, as each treatment condition deliberately built on the next, and as will be discussed shortly, the mechanism of measurement in each treatment condition precluded any reasonably known type of confounding variable from one treatment condition interfering with another treatment condition. Any influence from one treatment condition to another was deliberate and supportive of the stated primary and secondary hypothesis.

Description of Research Design

The study design utilized a within-subject design with three conditions: one pretest and two posttest conditions. After the intent of the study and the basic procedure to follow were explained, as well as addressing any questions or concerns, and a signed informed consent (Appendix A) was obtained, participants were then asked to read a standard eye chart and their vision was recorded. The first treatment condition was a measurement of the participant's vision prior to hypnosis.

The second treatment condition sought to address the secondary hypothesis regarding visual improvement via posthypnotic suggestion. This involved the measurement of vision after a posthypnotic suggestion to increase vision was given to the participant. The participant's vision was measured after hypnosis and after receiving a posthypnotic suggestion to improve vision. This entailed the participant being taken out of hypnosis and reading another variation of a standard eye chart.

The third condition addressed the primary research hypothesis regarding nonphysical sight. The third research condition existed after the participant was reintroduced to hypnosis and given an amnesia-induced posthypnotic suggestion creating a negative hallucination (rendering an object invisible) that was placed in front of a variation of a single-line chart. A negative hallucination is level 6 (L6) on the Arons hypnotic depth scale. The participant was then taken out of hypnosis and asked to read a unique variation of an eye chart that was directly behind a dry-erase board and impossible to see by normal visual perception.

Instruments of Measurement/Measurement Techniques

Two variations of a standard eye chart and a single-line eye chart, unique to each participant, were used to measure vision. A different variation of the standard eye chart was used in each of the first two treatment conditions and a single-line eye chart was used in the third treatment condition. At present, eye charts are considered a valid and reliable measurement of vision. The eye charts used were all read in descending fashion and increased in difficulty as the letters and numbers become smaller with each descending line. Typically, eye charts have a recorded vision that is measured with each descending line read on the eye chart and this is how they were utilized in this research study.

Previous Research and the Uniqueness of This Study

Regarding the second condition, there have been claims that hypnosis can enhance vision, as previously mentioned, going back to Braid (1843). Some of the studies have involved participants in the hypnotic state itself and some have been via posthypnotic suggestion. This study revisited the issue of hypnotic enhancement of vision. As the test for visual improvement answered the secondary research question, this study is not a comprehensive reexamination of hypnosis and posthypnotic suggestion and visual improvement; however, the findings of this study may facilitate future research in this area, as will be detailed in the discussion section of this paper.

Regarding the third condition of measuring for nonphysical sight, this is an area of research that has yet to be conducted. There does not appear to be any prior research seeking to measure the effect of altering subconscious beliefs to make an object invisible and then measure for nonphysical sight.

Participants

A total of 50 participants were utilized in this study. Participants filled out a short demographic questionnaire (see Appendix B). Ages ranged from 18 to 85. Of these, 13 were male, 37 were female. Regarding ethnicity, 44 self-identified as White, two identified as Hispanic, one identified as Filipino, one identified as Pacific Islander, one identified as Black and White, and one did not self-identify.

The total population of participants were tested for visual enhancement via hypnotic suggestion. Participants that read worse than 20/100 in treatment 1, or better than 20/16 in treatment 1 and treatment 2, were excluded from the eyesight data used in this study because these participants were off the scale of measurement, so to speak, and it was not possible to measure visual changes to eyesight. This resulted in 31 participants eligible to be included in the data set measuring for visual improvement. In this study, 10% of the participants were able to achieve a negative hallucination, which coincided with anecdotal estimates commonly stated by hypnotists on the percentage of people capable of a negative hallucination. The subset of total participants who were able to achieve L6, a negative hallucination, were measured for potential nonphysical sight. This subset of participants totaled five.

A convenience sample was used. Participants were solicited from faculty notifications to students at local universities and advertisements seeking participants in a research study measuring hypnotic depth level and hypnotic suggestion and visual improvement, in exchange for being taught a trigger for self-hypnosis (see Appendix C). A portion of the participants were offered nominal compensation for participation. The final 20 participants were paid either $20 or $50 in order to complete the research according to timeline guidelines.

Participants were required to be at least 18 years old. There was no maximum age requirement.

Materials

A private practice office with two chairs was used for the study (see Appendix D). The office building was located in an office complex with other professional offices. A private room at a spiritual retreat was also used, as was a conference room at a second private practice location. Two variations of a standard eye chart and multiple variations of a single-line eye chart, unique to each participant, were used (see Appendix E). A small erase board was used, as well as a small stand for the eye charts (see Appendixes F, G, and H).

Procedure

Informed consent. A benign form of deception was used in the experiment. Participants were told that the experiment was designed to measure hypnotic depth level and hypnotic suggestion and visual improvement. While that was true for the second treatment condition and the secondary hypothesis, it was not true regarding the third research condition and the primary hypothesis measuring nonphysical sight. Participants were given an informed consent disclosure

(Appendix A) advising them that deception may be used in the experiment and that they may withdraw from the research at any time.

Specific interventions. After participants signed an informed consent, a verbal explanation of the study and of hypnosis followed and any questions regarding the study and hypnosis were addressed. It was explained to participants that the purpose of the study was to measure hypnotic depth level and hypnotic suggestion in relation to visual improvement. Participants were told that the study was seeking to verify results from prior studies that have shown visual improvement with hypnosis and that have also shown that deeper states of hypnosis have shown greater effect with hypnotic suggestion. Participants were advised that they would be fractionalized, meaning that they would be taken in and out of hypnosis a few times to deepen their hypnotic state, and that their vision would be measured three times to see how much their vision improved with the deeper states of hypnosis.

After the intent of the study was explained and questions answered, participants were then asked to read a standard eye chart and their vision was recorded prior to hypnosis. It should be noted that the standard eye chart was turned around so the participants could only see the blank backside of the eye chart prior to reading it. The investigator was also blinded to the specific eye chart that was used in each session.

Participants were then hypnotized. A standard white light progressive relaxation induction with garden of the universe safe place imagery was utilized although these were loose guidelines, and varying of suggestions during the induction was allowed and tailored toward the specific reactions of the participant to the hypnotic suggestions. Participants were fractionalized (being taken in and out of hypnosis to deepen the hypnotic state) up to three or four times. The actual number of times each participant was fractionalized varied slightly as clinical discernment by the researcher was required to assess hypnotic depth level of the participant in the moment. Participants were given a special phrase via posthypnotic suggestion to reintroduce hypnosis each time the phrase was given; this was the means to achieve fractionalization.

Participants were provided a posthypnotic suggestion to improve their eyesight (Appendix I). Participants were then measured for visual improvement on a different variation of a standard eye chart. Again, the standard eye chart was turned around so the participants could only see the blank backside of the eye chart prior to reading it. Participants were asked to start reading at the same spot they started reading on the previous chart and then continue to read lines on the chart until unable to continue doing so. Measured eyesight on the standard eye chart was then recorded. After initial data collection it was determined to rotate the eye chart order with different participants in order to reduce the chance of any bias due to specific content of the eye charts that might impact the participant's responses. Hypnosis was reintroduced with the special phrase.

Hypnosis was then reintroduced. Participants were given an amnesia-induced posthypnotic suggestion (see Appendix I) creating a negative hallucination that a dry-erase board, which was placed in front of the eye chart, was invisible to them and that their conscious mind would have no memory of the suggestion; however, their subconscious mind would remember the suggestion and act on it.

While the participant was still hypnotized, an assistant to the researcher placed a dry-erase board directly in front of the standard eye chart and then exchanged the eye chart for the new single-line eye chart, which was randomly chosen from an envelope containing multiple single-line eye charts. The assistant then immediately left the room. The researcher/hypnotist kept his back to the dry-erase board that was blocking the eye chart until the assistant left the room. The placement and size of the dry-erase board made it impossible for the researcher or the participant to visually see the eye chart once it was behind the dry-erase board.

Participants were then tested again for eyesight, this time on the single-line eye chart. Participants were asked to read the single-line chart. For example, "I would like you to read the five letters on this single-line eye chart from left to right." After the participant read the line on the chart, or was incapable of doing so, the experiment ended and hypnosis was introduced for the purposes of providing a trigger to practice self-hypnosis. The results on the participant's performance on reading this line was recorded.

The reason the participant was only asked to read one single line of five letters was because the less the participants consciously thought about what they were doing, the less likely they would be to become aware of the negative hallucination. This could have occurred regarding increased difficulty in attempting to read the visually obstructed eye chart or by social cues by the experimenter, particularly if there was a measurable result for nonphysical sight. Awareness of the negative hallucination could potentially undermine the primary hypothesis regarding altering the subconscious belief in the object of visual obstruction and the potentiality of nonphysical sight. Future studies could investigate the longevity of the effect of nonphysical sight and include prolonged exposure to the state. This study simply sought to investigate the existence of nonphysical sight, not whether such a state or ability could be maintained.

Hypnosis was reintroduced via the special phrase, suggestions to countermand the negative hallucination were given, and a trigger to practice self-hypnosis was also given to the participant. Participants were then debriefed on the actual purpose of the study and how they performed.

Statistical analysis. The rationale for this approach was largely due to widespread acceptance of the validity and reliability of eye charts as an empirical measure of vision. In comparing the measured vision in treatment condition 1, in which vision was measured prior to hypnosis, and treatment condition 2, where vision was measured after hypnosis and a posthypnotic suggestion, a single-tailed paired sample t-test was used and a 5% significance level was established.

In the third treatment condition regarding the subset able to achieve a negative hallucination, a one-sample z-test was used, and hits or correctly stated letters were compared with probabilities based on a 5% significance level. With the subset of the population studied for nonphysical sight, a total of five participants were used.

A manila folder with data, including eye charts read and a recording of performance, was maintained for each participant. Notes on participants' idiosyncratic data were also recorded and mentioned in the discussion section of this paper if relevant. This included information such as if participants were able to achieve a negative hallucination or not, relevant to the third treatment condition, and also any relevant idiosyncratic information regarding the second treatment condition.

Ethical consideration. Benign deception was used in this study as participants were told that the study was measuring hypnotic depth level and visual improvement. Participants were not told that the primary purpose of the experiment was to test for nonphysical sight by altering subconscious belief. Temporary amnesia was also utilized. Misdirection and benign deception are inherent in hypnosis in the form of convincers and deepening techniques. In fact, the basis of the experiment was stage 6 on the Arons hypnotic depth scale commonly used by the National Guild of Hypnotists. Stage 6, which is a negative hallucination, inherently entails amnesia and deception regarding the suggestion. This is a technique used by thousands of hypnotists in depth testing and is considered safe by the National Guild of Hypnotists. Hypnotic suggestions countermanding the effect were not necessary as all participants able to achieve the negative hallucination were able to see the dry-erase board after the hypnosis session. Full disclosure was provided at the completion of the study and the researcher was available to address any concerns.

The hypnotherapist who conducted the research is a licensed psychotherapist and is a certified hypnotherapist who has met the requirements to practice therapeutic hypnosis in the state of Florida, which are considered stringent. Although the study was not necessarily therapeutic in nature, the researcher used clinical discernment and continuously evaluated participant safety throughout the procedure. While there are no known serious adverse reactions to hypnosis itself, if any adverse reactions occurred, the researcher was trained to deal with them and if necessary, had access to and could provide information on local mental health and medical resources. An informal mental health status exam was conducted to assure orientation x 4, person, place, time, and situation. During interview, participants were thus screened for signs of suicidality, hallucinations, delusions, major depression, and manic episodes, as well as other potential hazards or instability.

The researcher's clinical discernment was used to determine potential participants' exclusion from the research. This included but was not limited to any physical impairment, mental health condition, or cognitive impairment determined to pose a threat to the validity of the research, or the participant. One potential participant was excluded from participation due to a prior diagnosed serious mental health disorder. Another potential participant discontinued participation during the induction reportedly to emotional discomfort. In both incidences a debriefing was conducted, as well as a brief interview to assess and reduce potential emotional distress.

Limitations of the Study

In the test for improved vision in condition 2, one of the limitations for this study was that it may be measuring a temporary effect. There was also the potential of sensory cueing, whether the researcher influenced the participant's response to what was on the eye chart. This does not appear to have occurred as the researcher strived to be as neutral as possible, and a few participants actually showed a slight decrease in vision. However, the issue of potential sensory cueing may also be considered a limitation in this study. The ensuing results regarding visual improvement in condition 2 that reinforced prior studies may provide the basis for future research in this area. This future research could involve multiple hypnosis sessions over time and independent vision testing by an ophthalmologist not immediately after or during the hypnosis sessions, as well as optical examination looking for any biological changes to the eye prior to and after the treatment protocol. Similarly, condition 3, which was the test for nonphysical sight, also has potential limitations in that it may be measuring a temporary effect not transferable outside of the research condition and thus have limited external validity.

This design was chosen for practical reasons. A *between-subject* design would be an overly cumbersome undertaking as the required number of participants would be overly large for this study. Only a small number of participants were able to achieve a negative hallucination. This is the subset of participants being looked at regarding the primary hypothesis involving a negative hallucination. Thus, a small sample size poses limitation to the study, as will be discussed later.

Issues of Internal/External Validity

Issues of internal validity would be exemplified by one condition and the independent variable measured by that treatment condition, interfering with the independent variable being measured in another treatment condition in the same experiment. This issue appeared limited in this study. This issue was largely addressed by utilizing three different variations of an eye chart with each treatment condition. Two variations of a standard eye chart were alternated between treatments 1 and 2, and as stated, a single-line eye chart was used in treatment 3 that was unique to each participant. Thus, the memorization of the eye chart from one condition to another, which would be a confounding variable in the form of an internal validity issue, was eliminated. Other issues of internal validity were not relevant as each condition in this design built on the previous condition, which was supportive of the hypothesis; the previously mentioned fractionalization was necessary to deepen hypnosis and induce a negative hallucination in those capable of it. The participants and researcher were blinded to the eye charts in condition 3, as already discussed.

The first threat to internal validity in this experiment was the fact that a convenience sample was used. The study participants were not randomly chosen and did not represent a cross section of demographics. The research was conducted in a private practice hypnotherapy office, a private conference room, and a private room at a spiritual retreat. The study made use of opportunistic sampling; participants were solicited via emails to local university faculty who might have students interested in participating in the study, and others who responded to a solicitation seeking participants. Since this research experiment was largely dealing with potential human capabilities, there was an assumption that such abilities if they exist are universal to all humans. If that assumption was correct, then the use of a convenience sample should not interfere with research findings, although this is still an assumption lacking in empirical evidence. Since the study was mostly conducted in southwest Florida, a slightly older population was used. This may be the most plausible argument for a biological interference because human capabilities generally decrease with age. However, it is entirely plausible that the inverse effect of what is expected regarding age on human capability is possible, and it is entirely possible that declining physical capabilities could be fertile ground for the development of ESP, or in this case nonphysical sight, as a form of compensation. Still, it is not expected that there was a biological interference caused by the use of a convenience sample regarding potential ESP.

The ability of the hypnotist is certainly a factor that could enhance participant response to hypnotic suggestion or diminish it. This too seemed a minimal issue.

Another risk to internal validity for this research study was that participants could consciously become aware of the third condition regarding the negative hallucination. The potential threat of participants becoming consciously aware of the third condition was likely self-correcting. Participants not capable of achieving a hypnotic depth level where amnesia was able to be embedded into a posthypnotic suggestion were not likely to be able to achieve a negative hallucination. According to the NGH hypnotic depth levels, a posthypnotic suggestion is capable at the third depth level and a negative hallucination is the sixth and deepest depth level. This has also been verified by practical experience. Thus, these participants not capable of an amnesia-induced posthypnotic suggestion were not included in the subset of people who achieved a negative hallucination that was measured for nonphysical sight. The greater threat of conscious awareness to the negative hallucination would likely come from picking up a social cue from the experimenter regarding the uniqueness of the condition, or simply that the participant becomes aware of the uniqueness of the condition the longer that they are in it. This was addressed by brevity in the third condition.

Participants unable to achieve a negative hallucination, who became aware of the dry-erase board shielding the chart in the third condition, and who also attempted to intuit the letters, were included as a unique subset being measured for nonphysical sight; this will be addressed in the results section. Most participants who did not achieve a negative hallucination did not attempt to intuit any letters.

External validity, which is the ability to generalize the experimental results outside of the experimental condition, was jeopardized by using a convenience sample although, since the effect being measured was a biological capability as stated, this seemed not a high concern. The greater issue to external validity regarding the third condition was the potential inability to create the effect outside of the experimental design, as the design was specifically measuring subconscious beliefs below the screen of consciousness. Regarding the second condition, or the test for visual improvement, external validity may have been an issue, as this study was not measuring long-term effects and was only examining an immediate effect on improved vision.

Chapter 4: Results

A total of 50 participants were utilized in this study. Ages ranged from 18 to 85. Of these, 13 were male and 37 were female. Regarding ethnicity, 44 self-identified as White, two identified as Hispanic, one identified as Filipino, one identified as Pacific Islander, one identified as Black and White, and one did not self-identify. All participants were tested for vision before and after hypnosis. Thirty-one participants saw an increase in vision after hypnosis. Five participants were able to achieve a negative hallucination and these L6 participants were tested for nonphysical sight. An unexpected group of nine non-L6 participants emerged during the study who were able to see the dry-erase board yet still attempted to read the letters shielded by the dry-erase board, and as a result, were also tested for nonphysical sight.

The following results, although preliminary and tentative, did support the primary hypothesis that removing the subconscious belief in an object of visual obstruction would remove the limitations on perception and that nonphysical sight is possible. The secondary hypothesis that enhancing the subconscious belief in visual ability would result in improved vision was also supported. There did not appear to be any correlation to demographics of any kind and performance in either test.

Nonphysical Sight

Five L6 and nine non-L6 participants were tested under hypnosis for nonphysical sight using a single trial on which they were asked to identify five letters hidden behind a white dry-erase board. With 26 letters in the alphabet, the probability of identifying any given letter correctly was $1/26 = .038$. With each participant given five letters, the number of letters that each participant should have identified by chance is $.038 \times 5 = 0.19$ letter. In the L6 sample, five participants received 25 letters, so chance performance would be $3.8\% \times 25 = 0.95$ letter. In the non-L6 sample, nine participants received 45 letters, so chance performance would be 3.8% x 45 = 1.71 letters. With 14 participants in the combined samples, 70 letters were presented and chance performance would be 3.8% x 70 = 2.66 letters. Chance and achieved levels of performance on the nonphysical sight test are summarized in Table 1 for the study's five L6 participants, nine non-L6 participants, and the combined samples of 14 participants. Also shown in that table are the results of one-sample z-tests for sample proportions used to evaluate differences between achieved and chance levels of performance in each sample.

Table 1

Chance and Achieved Accuracy on the Nonphysical Vision Test in the L6 Sample, Non-L6 Sample, and Combined Samples With Results of z-Tests for Sample Proportions

Sample	Letters Presented	Chance Accuracy		Achieved Accuracy		Significance		
		% Identified	Number Identified	Number Identified	% Identified	z	p	d
L6 ($n = 5$)	25	3.8%	0.95	7	28.0%	2.83	.002	1.270
Non-L6 ($n = 9$)	45	3.8%	1.49	6	13.3%	1.49	.068	0.497
Combined ($N = 14$)	70	3.8%	2.66	13	18.6%	2.90	.002	0.775

Note. All significance levels (p) are one-tailed.

With this in mind, results were evaluated first for the five L6 participants, then the nine non-L6 participants, and then the combined sample of 14 L6 and non-L6 participants, and finally a comparison between the two groups.

Nonphysical sight among L6 participants. As explained above, each of the five L6 participants was expected by chance to identify 0.19 letters. Collectively, the five L6 participants were expected by chance to identify 5 x .19 = .95 letters. In fact, the L6 participants identified seven letters correctly. The performance of the L6 participants was evaluated against chance using a one-sample z-test for a sample proportion. The percentage of letters identified by the five L6 participants (7/25 = 28.0%) was significantly greater than would be expected by chance (0.95/25 = 3.8%), $z = 2.83$, $p = .002$ (one-tailed). A one-tailed test was used because the research hypothesis was that participants would identify *more* letters than chance would predict, not *fewer* letters. G*Power software Version 3.1.9.2 (Faul, Erdfelder, Lang, & Buchner, 2007) application for the one-sample t-test was used to calculate Cohen's d, a measure of effect strength. In this calculation, the proportion of letters identified correctly by the L6 sample (.280) was treated as the sample mean, and the proportion of letters expected to be identified correctly by chance (.038) was treated as the population mean. Treating proportions as means is appropriate because the mean of a collection of binary data (e.g., 0 = a letter was not identified correctly and 1 = a letter was identified correctly) is equal to the proportion of 1s; thus, a proportion is a mean. When the data are binary, the standard deviation σ is equal to $\sqrt{pq}$, where p = the proportion of 1s and q = the proportion of 0s (or 1-p). Thus, in calculating effect strength, the population standard deviation σ was set equal to $\sqrt{pq}$, where p = the proportion of letters one would expect to see identified accurately by chance and $q = 1 - p$: $\sigma = \sqrt{(.038)(.962)} = .191$. With those parameters, the value of Cohen's $d = 1.27$, which is a very strong effect by Cohen's (1988) standards. The strength of the effect is obvious to the naked eye as well. The L6 sample identified letters correctly (28%) at more than seven times the rate one would expect by chance (3.8%; Cohen, 1988).

Despite the strength of the effect and its statistical significance, caution should be exercised in interpreting this analysis of nonphysical sight among L6 participants due the inherent instability of any statistical analysis based on such a small sample. The addition or deletion of even a small number of cases could change the outcome of the analysis entirely. Because of the instability of statistical analyses of small samples, all of the findings of this study, and especially this finding, should be taken as suggestive, not definitive.

Nonphysical sight among non-L6 participants. The nonphysical sight performance of participants in the non-L6 group was also evaluated against chance using a one-sample z-test for a sample proportion. Collectively, the nine non-L6 participants identified six letters out of 45 presented (13.3%), while chance would predict 9 x .19 = 1.71 letters (or as a percentage, 1.71/45 = 3.8%). Although non-L6 participants identified more letters than was predicted by chance, the finding did not reach statistical significance: $z = 1.49$, $p = .068$ (one-tailed), $d = 0.497$. Although this effect was of medium strength, the small sample size involved prevented it from reaching statistical significance.

Nonphysical sight among L6 and non-L6 participants combined. The nonphysical sight performance of the combined L6 and non-L6 samples was also evaluated. These 14 participants were collectively presented with 70 letters. By chance, it would be expected that they would correctly identify 14 x .19 = 2.66 letters (or as a percentage, 2.66/70 = 3.8%). Collectively, the 14 L6 and non-L6 participants actually identified 13 letters (or as a percentage, 13/70 = 18.6%). Nonphysical sight performance in the combined L6 and non-L6 samples was significantly above chance: $z = 2.90$, $p = .002$ (one-tailed), $d = 0.775$. The effect was strong, but not exceptionally strong, by Cohen's (1988) standards, but was able to reach statistical significance by virtue of the somewhat larger combined sample size, $N = 14$ (Cohen, 1988).

Between-group comparison of nonphysical sight among L6 versus non-L6 participants. Table 2 summarizes chance and achieved levels of performance on the nonphysical sight test for a between-group comparison of the L6 and non-L6 samples. MedCalc software was used to perform the one-sample proportion tests described above, but MedCalc does not provide an online calculator to evaluate the difference between two independent sample proportions. Such a test is offered, however, by Vassar University. Their software was used to perform a between-group comparison of the percentages of letters identified correctly by participants in the L6 and non-L6 samples.

Table 2

Chance and Achieved Accuracy on the Nonphysical Vision Test in the L6 Sample and Non-L6 Sample and Results of a z-Test Comparison of Two Independent Proportions

	Samples		Significance		
	L6 ($n = 5$)	Non-L6 ($n = 9$)	z	p	d
Chance Accuracy	3.8%	3.8%			
Achieved Accuracy	28.0%	13.3%	1.51	.065	0.369

Note. The reported significance level (p) is one-tailed.

Collectively, the five L6 participants had the opportunity to identify 25 letters (five letters for each of the five L6 participants). Of these 25 letters, L6 participants identified seven letters (28.0% accuracy). Collectively, the nine non-L6 participants had the opportunity to identify 45 letters (five letters for each of the nine non-L6 participants). Of these 45 letters, non-L6 participants identified six letters (13.3% accuracy).

The between-group difference in these percentages was in the expected direction, with L6 participants identifying more letters than non-L6 participants, but did not reach statistical significance, $z = 1.51$, $p = .065$ (one-tailed). The G*Power application for the independent-samples *t*-test was used to calculate Cohen's *d* for this analysis. In that analysis, the proportions of letters identified correctly (p) in each sample (for L6, $p = .280$; for non-L6, $p = .133$) were treated as sample means, and sample standard deviations were calculated as $s = \sqrt{pq}$. With those parameters, Cohen's $d = 0.369$, a moderate strength effect that failed to reach significance due to the small samples that were involved in the comparison.

Posthypnotic Enhancement of Visual Accuracy

After excluding 19 participants who displayed either exceptionally good or exceptionally poor vision at T1, 31 cases remained for a comparison of visual accuracy before (T1) and after (T2) receiving a posthypnotic suggestion for enhanced vision. Table 3 provides descriptive statistics on the visual acuity dependent variable before and following posthypnotic enhancement. Figure 1 plots visual acuity means with 95% confidence interval error bars.

Table 3

Visual Acuity Before and Following Posthypnotic Visual Enhancement With Results of Within-Subjects t-Test

	Before Enhancement	After Enhancement	t	Significance df p			d_z
Means (Std. Deviations)	49.23 (29.12)	36.13 (21.88)	4.75	30	< .001		0.86

Note: $N = 31$.

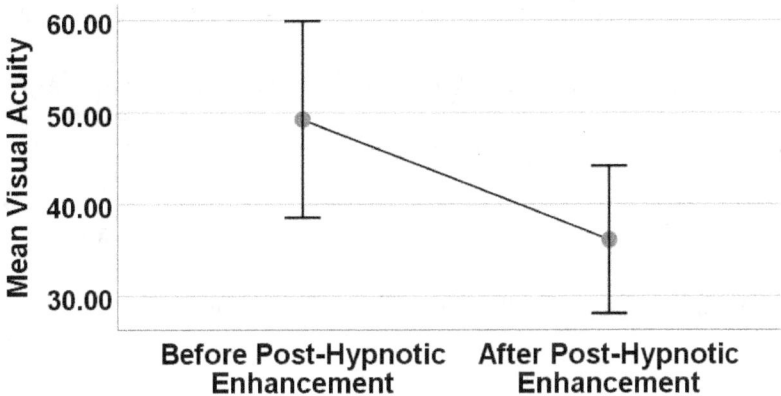

Figure 1. Mean visual acuity before and after posthypnotic enhancement. Error bars represent 95% confidence intervals for population means.

A paired-samples *t*-test from IBM SPSS (Version 25.0) was used to evaluate this within-subjects difference. The dependent variable in this test was the denominator of the visual acuity measure. Before performing the *t*-test, however, two statistical assumptions of the paired-samples *t*-test were evaluated. The first of these assumptions is that there should be no outliers (extreme values) among the difference scores (i.e., T2 – T1). This assumption was evaluated by standardizing the difference scores and screening for *z*-scores exceeding ± 3.30 ($p < .001$, two-tailed) as recommended by Tabachnick and Fidell (2013). No outliers were identified in this manner. The second assumption of the paired-samples *t*-test is that the difference scores should approximate a normal distribution. The distribution of T2 – T1 difference scores was evaluated for normality both visually and statistically. The visual evaluation of the distribution was accomplished by examining a frequency histogram of the difference scores. Statistical evaluations of the normality of the distribution were accomplished by testing values of skewness and kurtosis for significant deviations from 0 (the values of skewness and kurtosis associated with the normal curve), and also using the Shapiro-Wilk test of normality.

Figure 2 shows the frequency histogram of difference scores. The distribution provided a visual approximation to the normal curve, with more scores occurring toward the center of the score range than at the extremes. Measures of skewness = -0.48 and kurtosis = - 0.27 were standardized by dividing by their standard errors (skewness SE = .42; kurtosis SE = .82), and the resulting values of z were evaluated for significance against the normal distribution using the online calculator provided by Vassar University. Neither skewness, z = - 1.14, p = .254 (two-tailed), nor kurtosis, z = - 0.33, p = .741 (two-tailed), differed significantly from 0, the values of skewness and kurtosis that characterize the normal distribution. A Shapiro-Wilk test of the normality of the distribution of difference scores was also nonsignificant, $S\text{-}W$ = 0.94, df = 31, p = .080. It was concluded that the assumption of normally distributed difference scores was satisfied.

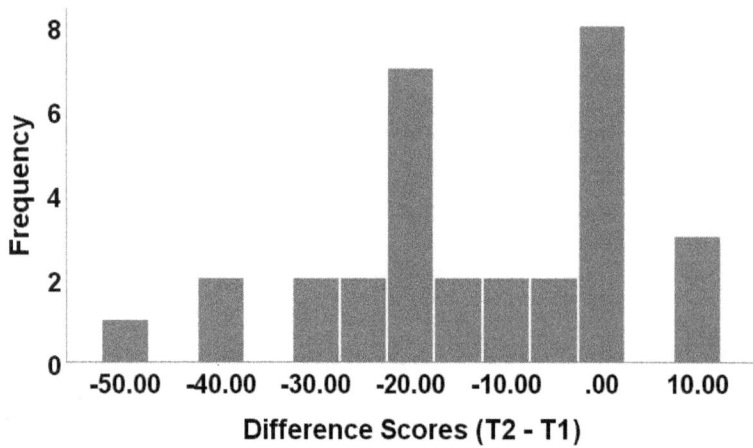

Figure 2. A frequency histogram showing the distribution of T2–T1 difference scores.

Having determined that both of the statistical assumptions of the paired-samples t-test were satisfied by the data, the t-test was performed. That test showed that vision after posthypnotic enhancement (M = 36.13, SD = 21.88) was significantly more accurate than before posthypnotic enhancement (M = 49.23, SD = 29.12), $t(30)$ = 4.75, p < .0005 (one-tailed).

Cohen's d_z measure of effect strength calculated using G*Power software found that the strength of the statistical effect was quite strong, $d_z = 0.85$ (Cohen, 1988). Out of 31 participants, 20 (64.5%) showed improvements from T1 to T2, eight (25.8%) showed no change, and three (9.7%) showed decreased visual accuracy.

Chapter 5: Discussion

The results of this study will be interpreted by first addressing the secondary hypothesis regarding the altering of subconscious beliefs utilizing hypnosis for the purposes of visual enhancement. This area of the research is explored first because the findings and implications are more straightforward. Secondly, the primary hypothesis asserting that the removal of a subconscious belief in an object of visual obstruction will remove the limitations on perception will be addressed. In each of these sections an explanation of the findings of this study will be followed by potential theories and then thoughts on future research and potential applications. Finally, a broad and general conclusion of the overall study will be broached.

Hypnosis and Visual Acuity

The results as stated were statistically significant regarding visual improvement from T1 to T2 after the intervention of hypnosis. The t-test showed that vision at T2 ($M = 36.13$, $SD = 21.88$) was significantly more accurate than at T1 ($M = 49.23$, $SD = 29.12$), $t(30) = 4.75$, $p < .0005$ (one-tailed). Cohen's dz measure of effect strength calculated using G*Power software version 3.1.9.2 found that the strength of the statistical effect was quite strong, $dz = 0.85$.

Findings and observations. The results of the test for visual acuity presented a variety of degrees of improvement in vision among participants. Out of 31 participants, 20 (64.5%) showed improvements from T1 to T2, eight (25.8%) showed no change, and three (9.7%) showed decreased visual accuracy. Subjectively, all participants reported enhanced vision, which included more vivid eyesight regarding both color and sharpness or contrast and a general brightness.

It is likely that the limits of the eye chart, which started at 20/100 and ended at 20/16, had an effect of underrepresenting the significance level of the visual improvement, as many of those excluded from the eventual analysis likely improved in vision. For instance, some participants who read 20/16 may have been able to read 20/10 after the hypnotic intervention. There were also participants reading worse than 20/100, which was the top end of the eye chart, and read 20/100 afterward, which also had to be excluded because it was not measurable.

It should be noted that the plastic eye charts used were standard eye charts; however, due to the fact that both eyes were measured at the same time, participants appeared to often read the first eye chart with greater visual acuity measured than they previously thought capable. It is actually possible that there may have been an indirect waking hypnotic suggestion created by the context of going to a hypnotist and participating in a hypnotic experiment measuring visual improvement, although it is more likely an effect of measuring both eyes simultaneously, resulting in one eye compensating for the other. This may have led to a greater number of participants being excluded from the hypnosis and visual acuity aspect of this study.

In the case of the three participants who actually decreased mildly in eyesight after hypnosis, this appears likely to be the result of not allowing enough time for the participants' eyes to adjust to the light after exiting a deep state of hypnosis. As the study went on, when a participant appeared to be struggling reading a line that they read prior to hypnosis, the researcher instructed them to blink and provided suggestions that their eyesight would clear, and this appeared effective.

Of those who saw visual improvement measured by reading the eye chart, the greatest increase in vision was from 20/80 to 20/30. Five participants increased in vision to 20/16, which was the best vision possible to measure by the eye chart. Of these, two participants read 20/40 before hypnosis and 20/16 after hypnosis, representing the largest increase of the participants who ended up reading 20/16.

Theories explaining effect. The temptation may be to explain away what are very significant results statistically by looking for solutions outside of hypnotic suggestion. Some may simply seek to explain these results by crediting relaxation as the cause of improved vision. One critique of studies involving hypnosis and increased visual acuity, as already mentioned, is that hypnosis may increase memorization, cognitive functions, and perceptual learning, resulting in a temporary improvement of vision (Raz et al., 2004).

The use of two different versions of a standard eye chart in this study seemed to address the issue of memorization. This study did not look at long-term effects of hypnosis and improved eyesight; this issue will be discussed shortly regarding suggested future research. It is possible that the effect of hypnosis and improved eyesight may be a temporary effect. Still, there are likely multiple explanations. While this research was a quantitative study, processes behind the mechanism of changes were not studied. The independent variable in the form of a hypnotic intervention was introduced and the dependent variable of changes to vision were measured. As stated, the changes to the independent variable were significant.

Given the body of research highlighted in the literature review, as well as an understanding of the basic compounding of suggestion and its increasing effect before, during, and after hypnosis, the possibility that the hypnotic state and hypnotic suggestion may in fact make biological changes resulting in increased vision, or simply allow an individual the ability to fully utilize current biological capabilities, should not be dismissed. Is the effect permanent or temporary? The answer may be that it depends. The permanency of hypnotic suggestion and visual improvement may depend on the belief, expectation, and motivation of the person being hypnotized. As has already been mentioned in the literature review, hypnosis alters subconscious beliefs by bypassing an individual's critical factor or conscious thought processes. It may very well be that the reconditioning of subconscious beliefs in many cases requires repetition. If we again consider hypnosis as a form of subconscious conditioning rather than relying on the computer programming metaphor, the idea that one hypnosis session should be able to make lasting change in the form of visual improvement after one session seems less plausible for most people. Most people have had a lifetime of conditioning regarding dependence on corrective lenses in the form of social confirmation, media, and prior experience. Expecting one session of hypnosis to permanently correct or improve vision is akin to expecting to get into top physical condition after one day of exercise that followed decades of physical neglect.

With this understanding, even if a hypnosis session does condition new biological changes, which could be considered behavioral changes on the micro level, such conditioning may require a reapplication of conditioning. For example, lutein has been shown to be important to visual development and function, especially the retina (Mares, 2016). If the consumption of lutein were discontinued, whether in the diet or in the form of supplements, and as a result its effect discontinued, would the biological effect be denied? Unlike a dietary supplement, the use of hypnosis may not be needed forever to see a continued effect. The cementing of the subconscious beliefs through hypnotic suggestion may require some degree of repetition in most cases, however.

This current research did not target the biology of the eye in the form of specific suggestions because such suggestions may require time to allow physical processes to start changing in the eye. The suggestions in this study were essentially direct regarding improved eyesight and requiring an immediate effect. Considering the statistical significance of the results, even if temporary, visual changes are likely the results of biological changes. The fact that such changes were instantaneous is noteworthy.

Future research. With the above in mind, the direction for potential future research is clear, as it is necessary. Future research involving the use of hypnosis for the purposes of visual improvement should involve multiple sessions, the targeting of biological systems in the eye, and biological measurements before and after the study. A comprehensive study of this nature at this date is necessary, as current and prior studies have been limited.

A study of this kind would ideally involve an ophthalmologist who would test for eyesight at the commencement of the study and then at its conclusion after the hypnotic intervention. The participating ophthalmologist would also ideally take a series of pictures and scans of the eyes before and after the study. These would be two objective measurements of effectual as well as biological changes. The proposed study should be conducted over a suitable period of time, preferably utilizing a hypnosis session once a week over 6 to 12 weeks. The use of a control group would also be ideal. Although standard procedures in eye exams do not consider the significance of sensory cueing on the part of the clinician, a protocol of this nature would address potential study limitation issues of sensory contamination as the researcher would be blinded to the eye charts, which was not fully the case in this study. The issue of whether a temporary or permanent effect is being observed would also be addressed with repetitive treatments over a longer period of time.

The hypnosis itself can be conducted in a private room at the ophthalmologist's office, although ideally, it would be conducted separately at a hypnotist's or hypnotherapist's office to avoid any form of indirect suggestions by staff that would potentially undermine the purpose. Asking innocent questions that possess indirect suggestions and embedded commands may undermine a session that just occurred when the participant is still highly suggestible. For example, asking, "Did it go well?" contains the indirect suggestion and embedded command that it could have gone well but also poorly. It would be best to avoid these potential confounding variables.

Another area of research that could follow a similar protocol may be to target those with chronic eye diseases such as macular degeneration. In this case, either improvement or slowing the progression of the disease could be compared to a control group.

Potential application. Most hypnotists are not licensed therapists. The profession of consulting hypnotism is unlicensed and has a limited scope of practice, depending on the state. If the results of future research supported the viability of hypnosis as a long-term effective strategy for visual improvement and maintaining eye health, the certifying of paramedical staff in hypnosis may enhance a private practice ophthalmology group, and eventually the ability to bill insurance for such services would follow. When dealing with issues of eye diseases, there is a potential for hypnosis to be added to the ophthalmologist's toolbox, especially for patients who struggle with adverse effects from medications or seek natural alternatives. Even if the hypnosis services are not provided at the ophthalmologist's office, the ophthalmologist could refer with confidence.

Hypnosis and Nonphysical Sight

The percentage of letters identified by the five L6 participants was significantly greater than would be expected by chance, $z = 2.83$, $p = .002$ (one-tailed). The value of Cohen's $d = 1.27$, which is a very strong effect size. Non-L6 participants identified more letters than was predicted by chance, although this group did not reach statistical significance, $z = 1.49$, $p = .068$ (one-tailed); $d = 0.497$. Although this effect was of medium strength, the small sample size involved prevented it from reaching statistical significance. The combined L6 and non-L6 samples was significantly above chance, $z = 2.90$, $p = .002$ (one-tailed); $d = 0.775$. The effect was strong, but not exceptionally strong, by Cohen's (1988) standards, but was able to reach statistical significance by virtue of the somewhat larger combined sample size, $N = 14$. The between-group difference in these percentages was in the expected direction, with L6 participants identifying more letters than non-L6 participants, but did not reach statistical significance, $z = 1.51$, $p = .065$ (one-tailed). Cohen's $d = 0.369$, a moderate strength effect that failed to reach significance due to the small samples that were involved in the comparison.

Findings and observations. There was a clear distinction observable between the L6 and non-L6 participants. L6 participants, when instructed to read the five letters shielded by the dry-erase board, did so quickly and easily without more than a couple of seconds' hesitation before stating the letters. Non-L6 participants had a much longer delayed response and appeared confused or strained before reading the letters. These visually observable differences to the researcher were verified afterward when debriefing the participants. While most non-L6 participants did not attempt to intuit letters, some did, and as a result an unexpected non-L6 group was created.

At the start of this research there was also some uncertainty as to the exact number of L6 participants that could be expected to emerge from the overall pool of participants. Numbers between 10% to 20% are often given by clinicians regarding the potential percentage of the population capable of a negative hallucination. It was the hope of this researcher to achieve greater than 20% of the participants in this study reaching L6. That did not occur and this research supported 10% as the approximate percentage of the population capable of reaching L6. This study may be the first quantifiable evidence that 10% of the population is capable of a negative hallucination. It should be noted that this is based on one session. It is possible that a greater percentage of the population may obtain L6 with repeated sessions.

L6 on the Arons scale for hypnotic depth was used as a basis for this study's exploration into the potentiality of nonphysical sight. The Arons scale of hypnotic depth, like all hypnotic depth scales, should be viewed as a guide and not rigidly, as the experience of hypnosis and various trance levels is very subjective and individualistic. On the surface, it would certainly appear that each level on the scale is deeper than the previous; however, several participants in this study appeared, based on physiology, to be in very deep states of hypnosis, but did not achieve L6.

It is also noteworthy that Elman (1964), in the 1940s through the 1960s, while training thousands of medical doctors, including psychiatrists and dentists, in clinical hypnosis, routinely hypnotized six or eight people at a time, inducing the Esdaile state, formerly called the coma state. This state was named after James Esdaile (1846), who performed thousands of serious surgeries using the state while hypnosis was still called mesmerism. This hypnotic state is characterized by a general anesthesia that occurs without suggestion, as well as a waxy-like catatonic state, and while the participant can respond to mental suggestion, he or she will not respond to physical suggestions due to a desire not to interrupt the euphoric state.

Based on the Esdaile state, which is considered the deepest state of hypnosis possible, and these observations regarding participants apparently in deep states of hypnosis, yet still unable to achieve L6, further exploration into L6 looking at brain wave activity and brain engagement of different regions of the brain are warranted. It is possible that L6 may require a suitable hypnotic depth, but it may also rely on the interaction and correlation of regions of the brain and the sequencing of such an interaction.

Another observation in this study was that it is possible to achieve level five (L5), which is a positive hallucination, and L6, which of course is a negative hallucination, at the same time.

After receiving the suggestion that the dry-erase board would be invisible, one L6 participant who named two letters reported afterward when being debriefed that he hallucinated a large dry-erase board and that he saw through it to see the letters. The researcher did not specify that the dry-erase board was small, which it was, so the participant imagined a large dry-erase board that is typically used in presentations. This ability to achieve both L5 and L6 simultaneously was previously unknown to the researcher and may be a novel discovery.

There were several non-L6 participants who did not state letters; however, when debriefed afterward, they reported that they were starting to see grey lettering bleeding through the dry-erase board. It is possible that these participants were beginning to achieve either L5 or L6. The emergence of these letters could have been either a positive hallucination or a negative hallucination. Exploring some of these idiosyncrasies in the data is helpful in conveying the dynamic and individualistic experience of hypnosis or trance states. Hypnotic or trance ability is much like athletics. Individuals have a natural propensity although with practice, most can become proficient. This issue will be touched on again shortly as future applications of these results are explored.

The actual performance results of each group in this study did support the hypothesis that removing the subconscious belief in an object of visual obstruction would remove the limitations on perception. The L6 group was small, only containing five participants, so these findings of evidence in support of nonphysical sight must be considered preliminary. Still, the effect was strong. There were also noted differences between the L6 and non-L6 groups tested for nonphysical sight. While this difference did not achieve statistical significance, it did support the hypothesis. The combined group of L6 and non-L6 participants totaled 14 and did achieve strong statistical significance when tested for nonphysical sight.

Theories explaining the effect. We can only speculate as to the mechanisms involved in the observed effect. As previously stated, this study was quantifiable since it focused on observable testable effects; however, the mechanisms and processes involved were not studied as the use of brain scans and other biological measurements were not utilized. Even if these measurements were utilized, there is still the uncomfortable acknowledgment that these measurements may be the effects, not the causes, because a suggestion is intangible. Therefore, we will speculate with these intangibles in mind.

When the difference between the L6 and non-L6 group is considered, the issue of the strength of the subconscious belief should be examined. While this research does support the hypothesis that removing the subconscious belief in an object of visual obstruction removed limitations on perception supporting the concept of nonphysical sight, there may be multiple viable explanations for the phenomenon.

Examined through the lens of the compounding of suggestion utilized in hypnosis, the creation of a negative hallucination of the L6 group could be considered as an amplification of the belief that one can see through an object of visual obstruction. The non-L6 participants who responded to the suggestion of being able to see through or around the object of visual obstruction were for the most part responding spontaneously to this suggestion to see through or around the object of obstruction, even though they still saw the object of visual obstruction.

These non-L6 participants did score better than chance although, as stated, did not achieve statistical significance. The explanation of strong statistically significant results for the L6 group compared to the non-L6 group may potentially be due to the belief negating the object of visual obstruction amplifying or removing a barrier to the belief of seeing through or around the object of obstruction. All L6 participants also achieved the temporary amnesia suggestion that was applied to the suggestion that the dry-erase board would be invisible and that they would be able to see through or around it. When they were prompted to read five large letters, these participants were not restricted by any conscious beliefs that they should not be able to read the letters. Contrastingly, the non-L6 participants saw the dry-erase board; however, most of this group that attempted to intuit letters reported that they either saw letters in their mind or that the letters just came to them.

These findings in themselves raise some interesting questions about the use of conscious amnesia-induced posthypnotic suggestions to enhance psychic ability in general. Conscious amnesia is often induced clinically to reduce self-sabotage regarding suggestions for behavioral changes. Would this strategy enhance psychic ability by blocking limiting beliefs in such an ability? It appears very plausible, given the specificity of the type of ESP that we are calling nonphysical sight, that a more general exploration of psychic phenomena is warranted.

It was speculated in the previous literature review that one basis for this study could be the existence of perceptual fields, and that such fields could operate in a similar fashion to magnetic fields in that they could go through or around an object, just as a magnetic field can exert influence through paper or cardboard. These preliminary findings with the L6 group do support that premise; however, again we observed effects but not the actual mechanism. At this time, there is not a way to measure hypothesized perceptual fields.

Humans certainly have attempted to see or intuit objects behind other objects or out of sight. The ability to negate the belief and perception of an object of visual obstruction may be unique to the human species and novel to this study. While speculative, if this is a new behavioral pattern of nature, its reinforcement may be necessary to condition a new ability.

Regardless of the mechanisms involved, the effect, if verified by future research, results from altering subconscious beliefs. Hypnosis, as has been argued, is the most effective method of altering subconscious beliefs. The potential impact on human potential is astounding if the altering of subconscious belief can enhance human capability. This is especially true regarding not only nonphysical sight, but also ESP in general. Up to this point, ESP was largely thought to be a quality that an individual possesses to a certain degree or not. If the subconscious belief is in fact the independent variable and ESP a dependent variable, then this potential human ability can be enhanced.

Future research. As indicated, a follow-up study is warranted. These findings, although statistically significant, must still be considered preliminary because of the small sample size. This research has established a benchmark that 10% of the population can achieve L6. Therefore, a follow-up study should be designed as follows. A pool of at least 300, but preferably 500, potential participants should be sought. Of this pool of participants, hypnotic depth testing should be conducted, and an expected 10% sample of L6 participants obtained from this group should be invited back to participate in the research. The same protocol used in this study should then be followed with the 30 or 50 participants. It would also be preferable to use several hypnotists in various locations conducting research with participants.

If the results of this larger study are also statistically significant, future research could involve increased training, especially in the area of self-hypnosis, in obtaining the appropriate trance state. As already indicated, while a natural propensity may exist, hypnosis or trance ability is largely a learned skill. Typically, more hypnotizable people not only go into a deeper trance, they also tend to do so more quickly. The required depth level with training in self-hypnosis and prior conditioning may be achieved within a minute or two with practice. It may also be possible to improve on actual performance with practice, not only in inducing the appropriate hypnotic state, but also in actual performance on the task at hand.

Potential applications. Besides the desire to improve human capability in general, this potential ability to train and enhance nonphysical sight may have military applications. For instance, the ability to see or intuit what is on the other side of a door could literally save a life. There may also be potential medical applications in emergency situations if a clinician is capable of inducing the condition necessary for nonphysical sight. As already indicated, these techniques may also have an impact on other areas of ESP in general, which may have broader applications.

Conclusion

These study results must be considered preliminary. Regarding the study results on eyesight improvement, even with the small sample size, at a very minimum, hypnotic suggestion and altering subconscious belief appears to impact biological functioning, even if just temporarily. The potential with repetition to alter the actual biology of the eye itself seems very plausible given the body of evidence demonstrating hypnosis influencing biology. Due to the small sample size, the evidence for nonphysical sight, although statistically significant and demonstrating a strong effect size, is preliminary with very tentative findings.

Still, if hypnotic suggestion can alter biology and even enhance human capability, then the power of suggestion at all levels of society needs further investigation. For instance, does watching a movie with middle-aged characters wearing glasses increase the probability of needing glasses as one ages due to indirect suggestion? Does a pharmaceutical advertisement on television showing images of arteries clogging increase the likelihood of arteries clogging through direct suggestion via an already hypnotic medium of television?

Can perceived limits to human potential and development be removed? More broadly, what is the relationship between belief and the actual physical structure of the universe? This research was exploratory. As such it raises more questions than answers.

References

Abramowitz, E. G., Barak, Y., Ben-Avi, I., & Knobler, H. Y. (2008). Hypnotherapy in the treatment of chronic combat-related PTSD patients suffering from insomnia: A randomized, zolpidem-controlled clinical trial. *International Journal of Clinical and Experimental Hypnosis, 56*(3), 270-280. doi:10.1080/00207140802039672

Abramowitz, E. G., & Lichtenberg, P. (2009). Hypnotherapeutic olfactory conditioning (hoc): Case studies of needle phobia, panic disorder, and combat-induced PTSD. *International Journal of Clinical and Experimental Hypnosis, 57*(2), 184-197. doi:10.1080/00207140802665450

Ahmad, B., & Zaman, K. (2011). Alternatives to simply forgiving and forgetting: Comparing techniques in hypnosis, NLP and time line therapy™ in reducing the intensity of memories of stressful events. *Stress and Health, 27*(3), 241-250. doi:10.1002/smi.1351

Alladin, A., & Alibhai, A. (2007). Cognitive hypnotherapy for depression: An empirical investigation. *International Journal of Clinical and Experimental Hypnosis, 55*(2), 147-166. https://doi.org/10.1080/00207140601177897

Alvarado, C. S. (2014). Mediumship, psychical research, dissociation, and the powers of the subconscious mind. *Journal of Parapsychology, 78*(1), 98.

Anbar, R. D., & Slothower, M. P. (2006). Hypnosis for treatment of insomnia in school-age children: A retrospective chart review. *BMC Pediatrics, 6*(1), 23. doi:10.1186/1471-2431-6-23

Aronoff, G. M., Aronoff, S., & Peck, L. W. (1975). Hypnotherapy in the treatment of bronchial asthma. *Annals of Allergy, 34*(6), 356.

Attias, J., Shemesh, Z., Sohmer, H., Gold, S., Shoham, C., & Faraggi, D. (1993). Comparison between self-hypnosis, masking and attentiveness for alleviation of chronic tinnitus. *International Journal of Audiology, 32*(3), 205-212.

Bakke, A. C., Purtzer, M. Z., & Newton, P. (2002). The effect of hypnotic-guided imagery on psychological well-being and immune function in patients with prior breast cancer. *Journal of Psychosomatic Research, 53*(6), 1131-1137. https://doi.org/10.1016/S0022-3999(02)00409-9

Barabasz, A. F., & Barabasz, M. (2015). The new APA definition of hypnosis: Spontaneous hypnosis MIA. *American Journal of Clinical Hypnosis, 57*(4), 459-463. https://doi.org/10.1080/00029157.2015.1011507

Barber, T. X. (1978). Hypnosis, suggestions, and psychosomatic phenomena: A new look from the standpoint of recent experimental studies. *American Journal of Clinical Hypnosis, 1*, 13-27. https://doi.org/10.1080/00029157.1978.10403953

Barber, T. X., & Wilson, S. C. (1977). Hypnosis, suggestions, and altered states of consciousness: Experimental evaluation of the new cognitive-behavioral theory and the traditional trance-state theory of "hypnosis." *Annals of the New York Academy of Sciences, 296*(1), 34-47. doi:10.1111/j.1749-6632.1977.tb38159.x

Barrios, M. V., & Singer, J. L. (1981). The treatment of creative blocks: A comparison of waking imagery, hypnotic dream, and rational discussion techniques. *Imagination, Cognition and Personality, 1*(1), 89-109. https://doi.org/10.2190/69G4-6YCM-N11H-EEEW

Baruss, I., & Mossbridge, J. (2017). *Transcendent mind*. Washington, DC: American Psychological Association.

Ben-Zvi, Z., Spohn, W. A., Young, S. H., & Kattan, M. (1982). Hypnosis for exercise-induced asthma. *American Review of Respiratory Disease, 125*(4), 392. doi:10.1164/arrd.1982.125.4.392

Berger, M. M., Davadant, M., Marin, C., Wasserfallen, J. B., Pinget, C., Maravic, P., & Chiolero, R. L. (2010). Impact of a pain protocol including hypnosis in major burns. *Burns, 36*(5), 639-646. https://doi.org/10.1016/j.burns.2009.08.009

Braid, J. (1843). *Neurypnology; or, the rationale of nervous sleep, considered in relation with animal magnetism*. London, England: John Churchill.

Bryant, R. A., Moulds, M. L., Guthrie, R. M., & Nixon, R. D. (2005). The additive benefit of hypnosis and cognitive-behavioral therapy in treating acute stress disorder. *Journal of Consulting and Clinical Psychology, 73*(2), 334. doi:10.1037/0022-006X.73.2.334

Burnett, O. L. (2015). The religion in medicine: An exploration of healing through the examination of Asclepius and the Epidaurian Iamata. *Prandium: The Journal of Historical Studies at University of Toronto Mississauga, 4*(1), 1-7. Retrieved from http://jps.library.utoronto.ca/index.php/prandium/article/view/25694

Calvert, E. L., Houghton, L. A., Cooper, P., Morris, J., & Whorwell, P. J. (2002). Long-term improvement in functional dyspepsia using hypnotherapy. *Gastroenterology, 123*(6), 1778-1785. https://doi.org/10.1053/gast.2002.37071

Cardeña, E. (2005). The phenomenology of deep hypnosis: Quiescent and physically active. *International Journal of Clinical and Experimental Hypnosis, 53*(1), 37-59.

Cardeña, E. (2014). A call for an open, informed study of all aspects of consciousness. *Frontiers in Human Neuroscience, 8*, 17. https://doi.org/10.1080/00207140490914234

Cardeña, E., Marcusson-Clavertz, D., & Wasmuth, J. (2009). Hypnotizability and dissociation as predictors of performance in a precognition task: A pilot study. *Journal of Parapsychology, 73*(1), 138-155.

Cardeña, E., Svensson, C., & Hejdström, F. (2013). Hypnotic tape intervention ameliorates stress: A randomized, control study. *International Journal of Clinical and Experimental Hypnosis, 61*(2), 125-145. https://doi.org/10.1080/00207144.2013.753820

Carmody, T. P., Duncan, C., Simon, J. A., Solkowitz, S., Huggins, J., Lee, S., & Delucchi, K. (2008). Hypnosis for smoking cessation: A randomized trial. *Nicotine & Tobacco Research, 10*(5), 811-818. https://doi.org/10.1080/14622200802023833

Carter, C. (2010). *Science and the near death experience: How conscousness survives death.* Rochester, VT: Inner Traditions.

Castel, A., Pérez, M., Sala, J., Padrol, A., & Rull, M. (2007). Effect of hypnotic suggestion on fibromyalgic pain: Comparison between hypnosis and relaxation. *European Journal of Pain, 11*(4), 463-468.

Castel, A., Salvat, M., Sala, J., & Rull, M. (2009). Cognitive-behavioural group treatment with hypnosis: A randomized pilot trail in fibromyalgia. *Contemporary Hypnosis, 26*(1), 48-59. https://doi.org/10.1016/j.ejpain.2006.06.006

Catoire, P., Delaunay, L., Dannappel, T., Baracchini, D., Marcadet-Fredet, S., Moreau, O., & Marret, E. (2013). Hypnosis versus Diazepam for embryo transfer: A randomized controlled study. *American Journal of Clinical Hypnosis, 55*(4), 378-386. https://doi.org/10.1080/00029157.2012.74794

Cohen, J. (1988). *Statistical power analysis for the behavioral sciences* (2nd ed.). Hillsdale, NJ: Erlbaum.

Collison, D. R. (1975). Which asthmatic patients should be treated by hypnotherapy? *Medical Journal of Australia, 1*(25), 776-781. https://doi.org/10.5694/j.1326-5377.1975.tb111851.x

Conn, L., & Mott, T., Jr. (1984). Plethysmographic demonstration of rapid vasodilation by direct suggestion: A case of Raynaud's Disease treated by hypnosis. *American Journal of Clinical Hypnosis, 26*(3), 166-170. https://doi.org/10.1080/00029157.1984.10404158

Cordi, M. J., Hirsiger, S., Mérillat, S., & Rasch, B. (2015). Improving sleep and cognition by hypnotic suggestion in the elderly. *Neuropsychologia, 69*, 176-182. https://doi.org/10.1016/j.neuropsychologia.2015.02.001

Cordi, M., Rossier, L., & Rasch, B. (2018). Improving night-time sleep with hypnotic suggestions. *bioRxiv 277566* (preprint). https://doi.org/10.1101/277566

Cordi, M. J., Schlarb, A. A., & Rasch, B. (2014). Deepening sleep by hypnotic suggestion. *Sleep, 37*(6), 1143. https://doi.org/10.5665/sleep.3778

Corey Brown, D., & Corydon Hammond, D. (2007). Evidence-based clinical hypnosis for obstetrics, labor and delivery, and preterm labor. *International Journal of Clinical and Experimental Hypnosis, 55*(3), 355-371. https://doi.org/10.1080/00207140701338654

Coué, E. (1922). *Self mastery through conscious autosuggestion.* New York, NY: Malkan.

Craciun, B., Holdevici, I., & Craciun, A. (2012). The efficiency of Ericksonian hypnosis in diminishing stress and procrastination in patients with generalized anxiety disorder. *European Psychiatry, 27*(1), 1136. https://doi.org/10.1016/S0924-9338(12)75303-8

Cupal, D. D., & Brewer, B. W. (2001). Effects of relaxation and guided imagery on knee strength, reinjury anxiety, and pain following anterior cruciate ligament reconstruction. *Rehabilitation Psychology, 46*(1), 28. http://dx.doi.org/10.1037/0090-5550.46.1.28

Cyna, A. M., Andrew, M. I., & McAuliffe, G. L. (2006). Antenatal self-hypnosis for labour and childbirth: A pilot study. *Anaesthesia and Intensive Care, 34*(4), 464-469. https://doi.org/10.1177/0310057X0603400402

Dane, J. R. (1996). Hypnosis for pain and neuromuscular rehabilitation with multiple sclerosis: Case summary, literature review, and analysis of outcomes. *International Journal of Clinical and Experimental Hypnosis, 44*(3), 208-231. https://doi.org/10.1080/00207149608416084

Davison, G. C., & Singleton, L. (1967). A preliminary report of improved vision under hypnosis. *International Journal of Clinical and Experimental Hypnosis, 15*(2), 57-62. https://doi.org/10.1080/00207146708407509

Deabler, H. L., Fidel, E., Dillenkoffer, R. L., & Elder, S. T. (1973). The use of relaxation and hypnosis in lowering high blood pressure. *American Journal of Clinical Hypnosis, 16*(2), 75-83. https://doi.org/10.1080/00029157.1973.10403656

Decety, J. (1996). Do imagined and executed actions share the same neural substrate? *Cognitive Brain Research, 3*(2), 87-93. https://doi.org/10.1016/0926-6410(95)00033-X

Del Prete, G., & Tressoldi, P. E. (2005). Anomalous cognition in hypnagogic state with OBE induction: An experimental study. *Journal of Parapsychology, 69*(2), 329.

Derbyshire, S. W., Whalley, M. G., & Oakley, D. A. (2009). Fibromyalgia pain and its modulation by hypnotic and non-hypnotic suggestion: An fMRI analysis. *European Journal of Pain, 13*(5), 542-550.

Derbyshire, S. W., Whalley, M. G., Stenger, V. A., & Oakley, D. A. (2004). Cerebral activation during hypnotically induced and imagined pain. *NeuroImage, 23*(1), 392-401. doi:10.1016/j.ejpain.2008.06.010

Diamond, S. G., Davis, O. C., Schaechter, J. D., & Howe, R. D. (2006). Hypnosis for rehabilitation after stroke: Six case studies. *Contemporary Hypnosis, 23*(4), 173-180. https://doi.org/10.1002/ch.319

Dinges, D. F., Whitehouse, W. G., Orne, E. C., Bloom, P. B., Carlin, M. M., Bauer, N. K., & Orne, M. T. (1997). Self-hypnosis training as an adjunctive treatment in the management of pain associated with sickle cell disease. *International Journal of Clinical and Experimental Hypnosis, 45*(4), 417-432. doi:10.1080/00207149708416141

Doidge, N. (2007). *The brain that changes itself.* New York, NY: Penguin.

Donaldson, V. W. (2000). A clinical study of visualization on depressed white blood cell count in medical patients. *Applied Psychophysiology and Biofeedback, 25*(2), 117-128. http://dx.doi.org/10.1023/A:1009518925859

Dubin, L. L., & Shapiro, S. S. (1974). Use of hypnosis to facilitate dental extraction and hemostasis in a classic hemophiliac with a high antibody titer to factor VIII. *American Journal of Clinical Hypnosis, 17*(2), 79-83. doi:10.1080/00029157.1974.10403718

Eitner, S. W. (2006). Rapid induction of hypnosis by finger elongation: A brief communication. *International Journal of Clinical and Experimental Hypnosis, 54*(3), 245-262. doi:10.1080/00207140600689405

Elahi, Z., Boostani, R., & Motie Nasrabadi, A. (2012). Estimation of hypnosis susceptibility based on electroencephalogram signal features. *Scientia Iranica, 20*(3), 730-737. https://doi.org/10.1016/j.scient.2012.07.015

Elkins, G. R., Barabasz, A. F., Council, J. R., & Spiegel, D. (2015). Advancing research and practice: The revised APA Division 30 definition of hypnosis. *International Journal of Clinical and Experimental Hypnosis, 63*(1), 1-9. https://doi.org/10.1080/00207144.2014.961870

Elkins, G. R., Jensen, M. P., & Patterson, D. R. (2007). Hypnotherapy for the management of chronic pain. *International Journal of Clinical and Experimental Hypnosis, 55*(3), 275-287. https://doi.org/10.1080/00207140701338621

Elkins, G. R., Johnson, A., Fisher, W., Sliwinski, J., & Keith, T. Z. (2013). A pilot investigation of guided self-hypnosis in the treatment of hot flashes among postmenopausal women. *International Journal of Clinical and Experimental Hypnosis, 61*(3), 342-350. https://doi.org/10.1080/00207144.2013.784112

Elkins, G. R., Marcus, J., Bates, J., Hasan Rajab, M., & Cook, T. (2006). Intensive hypnotherapy for smoking cessation: A prospective study 1. *International Journal of Clinical and Experimental Hypnosis, 54*(3), 303-315. doi:10.1080/00207140600689512

Elkins, G. R., & Rajab, M. H. (2004). Clinical hypnosis for smoking cessation: Preliminary results of a three-session intervention. *International Journal of Clinical and Experimental Hypnosis, 52*(1), 73-91. doi:10.1076/iceh.52.1.73.23921

Elkins, G. R., Sliwinski, J., Bowers, J., & Encarnacion, E. (2013). Feasibility of clinical hypnosis for the treatment of Parkinson's disease: A case study. *International Journal of Clinical and Experimental Hypnosis, 61*(2), 172-182. https://doi.org/10.1080/00207144.2013.753829

Elman, D. (1964). *Hypnotherapy.* London, England: Westwood.

Eremin, O., Walker, M. B., Simpson, E., Heys, S. D., Ah-See, A. K., Hutcheon, A. W., & Walker, L. G. (2009). Immuno-modulatory effects of relaxation training and guided imagery in women with locally advanced breast cancer undergoing multimodality therapy: A randomised controlled trial. *The Breast, 18*(1), 17-25. https://doi.org/10.1016/j.breast.2008.09.002

Esdaile, J. (1846). *Mesmerism in India: And its practical application in surgery and medicine.* London, England: Longman, Brown, Green, & Longman.

Esdaile, J. (1852). *Natural and mesmeric clairvoyance.* London, England: Hippolyte Bailliere.

Facco, E., Pasquali, S., Zanette, G., & Casiglia, E. (2013). Hypnosis as sole anaesthesia for skin tumour removal in a patient with multiple chemical sensitivity. *Anaesthesia, 68*(9), 961-965. https://doi.org/10.1111/anae.12251

Faul, F., Erdfelder, E., Lang, A. G., & Buchner, A. (2007). G*Power 3: A flexible statistical power analysis program for the social, behavioral, and biomedical sciences. *Behavioral Research Methods, 39*, 175-191.

Faymonville, M. E., Mambourg, P. H., Joris, J., Vrijens, B., Fissette, J., Albert, A., & Lamy, M. (1997). Psychological approaches during conscious sedation. Hypnosis versus stress reducing strategies: a prospective randomized study. *Pain, 73*(3), 361-367. https://doi.org/10.1016/S0304-3959(97)00122-X

Fillmer, H. T. (1980). Improving reading performances through hypnosis. *Community College Review, 2*, 58-62. https://doi.org/10.1177/009155218100900211

Flore, L. D. (2014). Interest of hypnosis in cataract surgery, about 99 patients. *Investigative Ophthalmology & Visual Science, 55*(13), 2541.

Freedman, M., Binns, M., Gao, F., Holmes, M., Roseborough, A., Strother, S., & Ryan, J. D. (2018). Mind-matter interactions and the frontal lobes of the brain: A novel neurobiological model of psi inhibition. *Explore, 14*(1), 76-85. doi:10.1016/j.explore.2017.08.003

Freeman, R., Barabasz, A., Barabasz, M., & Warner, D. (2000). Hypnosis and distraction differ in their effects on cold pressor pains. *American Journal of Clinical Hypnosis, 43*(2), 137-148. doi:10.1080/00029157.2000.10404266

Fry, L., Mason, A. A., & Pearson, R. B. (1964). Effect of hypnosis on allergic skin responses in asthma and hay-fever. *British Medical Journal, 1*(5391), 1145-1148. doi:10.1136/bmj.1.5391.1145

Gajan, F., Pannetier, B., Cordier, A., Amstutz-Montadert, I., Dehesdin, D., & Marie, J. P. (2011). Role of hypnotherapy in the treatment of debilitating tinnitus. *Revue de laryngologie-otologie-rhinologie, 133*(3), 147.

Ganis, G., Thompson, W. L., & Kosslyn, S. M. (2004). Brain areas underlying visual mental imagery and visual perception: An fMRI study. *Cognitive Brain Research, 20*(2), 226-241. https://doi.org/10.1016/j.cogbrainres.2004.02.012

Ginandes, C., Brooks, P., Sando, W., Jones, C., & Aker, J. (2003). Can medical hypnosis accelerate post-surgical wound healing? Results of a clinical trial. *American Journal of Clinical Hypnosis, 45*(4), 333-351. doi:10.1080/00029157.2003.10403546

Ginandes, C. S., & Rosenthal, D. I. (1999). Using hypnosis to accelerate the healing of bone fractures: A randomized controlled pilot study. *Alternative Therapies in Health and Medicine, 5*(2), 67.

Goldfine, I. D., Abraira, C., Gruenewald, D., & Goldstein, M. S. (1970). Plasma insulin levels during imaginary food ingestion under hypnosis. *Proceedings of the Society for Experimental Biology and Medicine, 133*(1), 274-276. doi:10.3181/00379727-133-34454

Gonsalkorale, W. M., & Whorwell, P. J. (2005). Hypnotherapy in the treatment of irritable bowel syndrome. *European Journal of Gastroenterology & Hepatology, 17*(1), 15-20. doi:10.1097/00042737-200501000-00004

Grabowska, M. J. (1971). The effect of hypnosis and hypnotic suggestion on the blood flow in the extremities. *Polish Medical Journal, 10*(4), 1044-1051.

Graham, C., & Leibowitz, H. W. (1972). The effect of suggestion on visual acuity. *International Journal of Clinical and Experimental Hypnosis, 20*(3), 169-186. http://dx.doi.org/10.1080/00207147208409288

Gruner, H. (2010). The cult of Asclepius—the temples of medicine. *Medicina Interna Revista da Sociedade Portuguesa de Medicina Interna, 17*(2), 122.

Gur, R. C., & Reyher, J. (1976). Enhancement of creativity via free-imagery and hypnosis. *American Journal of Clinical Hypnosis, 18*(4), 237-249. https://doi.org/10.1080/00029157.1976.10403806

Guttman, K., & Ball, T. S. (2013). An unanticipated allergic reaction to a hypnotic suggestion for anesthesia: A brief communication and commentary. *International Journal of Clinical and Experimental Hypnosis, 61*(3), 336-341. https://doi.org/10.1080/00207144.2013.784100

Halsband, U., Mueller, S., Hinterberger, T., & Strickner, S. (2009). Plasticity changes in the brain in hypnosis and meditation. *Contemporary Hypnosis, 26*(4), 194-215. https://doi.org/10.1002/ch.386

Hammer, E. F. (1954). Post-hypnotic suggestion and test performance. *International Journal of Clinical and Experimental Hypnosis, 2*(3), 178-185. https://doi.org/10.1080/00207145408410053

Hammond, D. C. (2007). Review of the efficacy of clinical hypnosis with headaches and migraines. *International Journal of Clinical and Experimental Hypnosis, 55*(2), 207-219. https://doi.org/10.1080/00207140601177921

Hammond, D. C. (2010). Hypnosis in the treatment of anxiety and stress related disorders. *Expert Review of Neurotherapeutic, 10*(2), 263-273. https://doi.org/10.1586/ern.09.140

Harmon, T. M., Hynan, M. T., & Tyre, T. E. (1990). Improved obstetric outcomes using hypnotic analgesia and skill mastery combined with childbirth education. *Journal of Consulting and Clinical Psychology, 58*(5), 525. doi:10.1037/0022-006X.58.5.525

Hart, G. D. (1965). Asclepius, god of medicine. *Canadian Medical Association Journal, 92*(5), 232.

Harte, R. (1991). *Train the trainer hypnotism certification manual.* Merrimack, NH: National Guild of Hypnotists.

Hawkins, P., & Polemikos, N. (2002). Hypnosis treatment of sleeping problems in children experiencing loss. *Contemporary Hypnosis, 19*(1), 18-24. https://doi.org/10.1002/ch.236

Hoeft, F., Gabrieli, J. D., Whitfield-Gabrieli, S., Haas, B. W., Bammer, R., Menon, V., & Spiegel, D. (2012). Functional brain basis of hypnotizability. *Archives of General Psychiatry, 69*(10), 1064-1072. doi:10.1001/archgenpsychiatry.2011.2190

Horton-Hausknecht, J. R., Mitzdorf, U., & Melchart, D. (2000). The effect of hypnosis therapy on the symptoms and disease activity in rheumatoid arthritis. *Psychology & Health, 14*(6), 1089-1104. https://doi.org/10.1080/08870440008407369

James, T., Flores, L., & Schober, J. (2016). *Hypnosis: A comprehensive guide.* Bancyfelin, Carmarthen, Wales: Crown House.

James, W. (1902). *The varieties of religious experience.* New York, NY: Random House.

Jensen, M. P., Barber, J., Romano, J. M., Molton, I. R., Raichle, K. A., Osborne, T. L., & Patterson, D. R. (2009). A comparison of self-hypnosis versus progressive muscle relaxation in patients with multiple sclerosis and chronic pain. *International Journal of Clinical and Experimental Hypnosis, 57*(2), 198-221.

Jensen, M. P., McArthur, K. D., Barber, J., Hanley, M. A., Engel, J. M., Romano, J. M., & Patterson, D. R. (2006). Satisfaction with, and the beneficial side effects of, hypnotic analgesia. *International Journal of Clinical and Experimental Hypnosis, 54*(4), 432-447. https://doi.org/10.1080/00207140802665476

Jung, C. G. (1936). The concept of the collective unconscious. In G. Adler & R. F. Hull (Eds. & Trans.), *The collected works of C. G. Jung* (2nd ed., Vol. 9, Part 1, pp. 42-53). Princeton, NJ: Princeton University Press.

Kaminsky, D., Rosca, P., Budowski, D., Korin, Y., & Yakhnich, L. (2007). Group hypnosis treatment of drug addicts. *Harefuah, 147*(8-9), 679-683.

Kay, L. (1992). *The effects of hypnosis, relaxation, and suggestion on visual acuity* (Unpublished doctoral disssertation). California School of Professional Psychology, Oakland, CA.

Kirsch, I., & Lynn, S. J. (1995). Altered state of hypnosis: Changes in the theoretical landscape. *American Psychologist, 50*(10), 846-858.

Kirsch, I., Montgomery, G., & Sapirstein, G. (1995). Hypnosis as an adjunct to cognitive-behavioral psychotherapy: A meta-analysis. 214. *Journal of Consulting and Clinical Psychology, 2*, 214. doi:10.1037//0022-006X.63.2.214

Koe, G. G., & Oldridge, O. A. (1988). The effect of hypnotically induced suggestions on reading performance. *International Journal of Clinical and Experimental Hypnosis, 36*(4), 275-283. https://doi.org/10.1080/00207148808410518

Kohen, D. P., & Zajac, R. (2007). Self-hypnosis training for headaches in children and adolescents. *The Journal of Pediatrics, 150*(6), 635-639. https://doi.org/10.1016/j.jpeds.2007.02.014

Kool, S. (2015). The soother of evil pains: Asclepius and Freud. *Akroterion, 60*(1), 13-32. doi:10.7445/60-1-938

Kraft, D. (2012). Panic disorder without agoraphobia. A multimodal approach: Solution-focused therapy, hypnosis and psychodynamic psychotherapy. *Journal of Integrative Research, Counselling and Psychotherapy, 1*(1), 4-15.

Kraft, T., & Kraft, D. (2004). Creating a virtual reality in hypnosis: A case of driving phobia. *Contemporary Hypnosis, 21*(2), 79-85. https://doi.org/10.1002/ch.293

Lang, E. V., Benotsch, E. G., Fick, L. J., Lutgendorf, S., Berbaum, M. L., Berbaum, K. S., & Spiegel, D. (2000). Adjunctive non-pharmacological analgesia for invasive medical procedures: A randomised trial. *Lancet, 355*(9214), 1486-1490. https://doi.org/10.1016/S0140-6736(00)02162-0

Langer, E., Djikic, M., Pirson, M., Madenci, A., & Donohue, R. (2010). Believing is seeing using mindlessness (mindfully) to improve visual acuity. *Psychological Science, 21*(5), 661-666. https://doi.org/10.1177/0956797610366543

Levitas, E., Parmet, A., Lunenfeld, E. B., Burstein, E., Friger, M., & Potashnik, G. (2006). Impact of hypnosis during embryo transfer on the outcome of in vitro fertilization–embryo transfer: A case-control study. *Fertility and Sterility, 85*(5), 1404-1408. https://doi.org/10.1016/j.fertnstert.2005.10.035

Liossi, C., & Hatira, P. (1999). Clinical hypnosis versus cognitive behavioral training for pain management for pediatric cancer patients undergoing bone marrow aspirations. *International Journal of Clinical and Experimental Hypnosis, 47*(2), 104-116. https://doi.org/10.1080/00207149908410025

Liossi, C., & Hatira, P. (2003). Clinical hypnosis in the alleviation of procedure-related pain in pediatric oncology patients. *International Journal of Clinical and Experimental Hypnosis, 51*(1), 4-28. doi:10.1076/iceh.51.1.4.14064

Liossi, C., & White, P. (2001). Efficacy of clinical hypnosis in the enhancement of quality of life of terminally ill cancer patients. *Contemporary Hypnosis, 18*(3), 145-160. https://doi.org/10.1002/ch.228

Liossi, C., White, P., & Hatira, P. (2006). Randomized clinical trial of local anesthetic versus a combination of local anesthetic with self-hypnosis in the management of pediatric procedure-related pain. *Health Psychology, 25*(3), 307. http://dx.doi.org/10.1037/0278-6133.25.3.307

Lynn, S. J., Green, J. P., Kirsch, I., Capafons, A., Lilienfeld, S. O., Laurence, J. R., & Montgomery, G. H. (2015). Grounding hypnosis in science: The "new" APA division 30 definition of hypnosis as a step backward. *American Journal of Clinical Hypnosis, 54*(4), 390-401. https://doi.org/10.1080/00029157.2015.1011472

Machovec, F. J. (1979). The cult of Asklipios. *American Journal of Clinical Hypnosis, 22*(20), 85-90. https://doi.org/10.1080/00029157.1979.10403203

Madrid, A., Rostel, G., Pennington, D., & Murphy, D. (1995). Subjective assessment of allergy relief following group hypnosis and self-hypnosis: A preliminary study. *American Journal of Clinical Hypnosis, 38*(2), 80-86. https://doi.org/10.1080/00029157.1995.10403186

Maher-Loughnan, G. P. (1970). Hypnosis and autohypnosis for the treatment of asthma. *International Journal of Clinical and Experimental Hypnosis, 18*(1), 1-14. https://doi.org/10.1080/00207147008415898

Maher-Loughnan, G. P., Macdonald, N., Mason, A. A., & Fry, L. (1962). Controlled trial of hypnosis in the symptomatic treatment of asthma. *British Medical Journal, 2*(5301), 371-376. doi:10.1136/bmj.2.5301.371

Manganiello, A. J. (1984). A comparative study of hypnotherapy and psychotherapy in the treatment of methadone addicts. *American Journal of Clinical Hypnosis, 26*(4), 273-279. https://doi.org/10.1080/00029157.1984.10402575

Manganiello, A. J. (1986). Hypnotherapy in the rehabilitation of a stroke victim: A case study. *American Journal of Clinical Hypnosis, 29*(1), 64-68. https://doi.org/10.1080/00029157.1986.10402680

Mares, J. (2016). Lutein and zeaxanthin isomers in eye health and disease. *Annual Review of Nutrition, 36*, 571-602. doi:10.1146/annurev-nutr-071715-051110

Mason, A. A. (1952). Case of congenital ichthyosiform erythrodermia of brocq treated by hypnosis. *British Medical Journal, 2*(4781), 422-423. doi:10.1136/bmj.2.4781.422

McGeown, W. J., Mazzoni, G., Venneri, A., & Kirsch, I. (2009). Hypnotic induction decreases anterior default mode activity. *Consciousness and Cognition, 18*(4), 848-855. https://doi.org/10.1016/j.concog.2009.09.001

Mehl-Madrona, L. E. (2004). Hypnosis to facilitate uncomplicated birth. *American Journal of Clinical Hypnosis, 46*(4), 299-312. https://doi.org/10.1080/00029157.2004.10403614

Miller, S. D. (1989). Optical differences in cases of multiple personality disorder. *Journal of Nervous and Mental Disease, 177*(8), 480-486. http://dx.doi.org/10.1097/00005053-198908000-00005

Miller, V., & Whorwell, P. J. (2008). Treatment of inflammatory bowel disease: A role for hypnotherapy? *International Journal of Clinical and Experimental Hypnosis, 56*(3), 306-317. https://doi.org/10.1080/00207140802041884

Mirzamani, S. M., Bahrami, H., Moghtaderi, S., & Namegh, M. (2012). The effectiveness of hypnotherapy in treating depression, anxiety and sleep disturbance caused by subjective tinnitus. *Zahedan Journal of Research in Medical Sciences, 14*(9), 76-79.

Montgomery, G. H., David, D., Winkel, G., Silverstein, J. H., & Bovbjerg, D. H. (2002). The effectiveness of adjunctive hypnosis with surgical patients: A meta-analysis. *Anesthesia & Analgesia, 94*(6), 1639-1645. doi:10.1213/00000539-200206000-00052

Montgomery, G. H., DuHamel, K. N., & Redd, W. H. (2000). A meta-analysis of hypnotically induced analgesia: How effective is hypnosis? *International Journal of Clinical and Experimental Hypnosis, 48*(2), 138-153. https://doi.org/10.1080/00207140008410045

Montgomery, G. H., Weltz, C. R., Seltz, M., & Bovbjerg, D. H. (2002). Brief presurgery hypnosis reduces distress and pain in excisional breast biopsy patients. *International Journal of Clinical and Experimental Hypnosis, 50*(1), 17-32. https://doi.org/10.1080/00207140208410088

Moore, L. E., & Kaplan, J. Z. (1983). Hypnotically accelerated burn wound healing. *American Journal of Clinical Hypnosis, 26*(1), 16-19. https://doi.org/10.1080/00029157.1983.10404132

Müller, K., Bacht, K., Schramm, S., & Seitz, R. J. (2012). The facilitating effect of clinical hypnosis on motor imagery: An fMRI study. *Behavioural Brain Research, 23*(1), 164-169. https://doi.org/10.1016/j.bbr.2012.03.013

Nemeth, D., Janacsek, K., Polner, B., & Kovacs, Z. A. (2013). Boosting human learning by hypnosis. *Cerebral Cortex, 23*(4), 801-805. https://doi.org/10.1093/cercor/bhs068

Newmark, T. (2012). Cases in visualization for improved athletic performance psychiatric annals. *Psychiatric Annals, 42*(10), 385-387. https://doi.org/10.3928/00485713-20121003-07

Noble, S. (2002). The management of blood phobia and a hypersensitive gag reflex by hypnotherapy: A case report. *Dental Update, 29*(2), 70-74. https://doi.org/10.12968/denu.2002.29.2.70

Noll, R. B. (1994). Hypnotherapy for warts in children and adolescents. *Journal of Developmental & Behavioral Pediatrics, 15*(3), 170-173.

Page, S. J., Levine, P., Sisto, S., & Johnston, M. V. (2001). A randomized efficacy and feasibility study of imagery in acute stroke. *Clinical Rehabilitation, 15*(3), 233-240. https://doi.org/10.1191/026921501672063235

Panagiotidou, O. (2016). Religious healing and the Asclepius cult: A case of placebo effects. *Open Theology, 2*(1), 79-91. doi:10.1515/opth-2016-0006

Parra, A., & Argibay, J. C. (2013). A free-response ESP test in two hypnotic susceptibility groups: A pilot study. *Australian Journal of Parapsychology, 13*(1), 27.

Pates, J. (2013). The effects of hypnosis on an elite senior european tour golfer: A single-subject design. *International Journal of Clinical and Experimental Hypnosis, 61*(2), 193-204. https://doi.org/10.1080/00207144.2013.753831

Pates, J., Cummings, A., & Maynard, I. (2002). The effects of hypnosis on flow states and three-point shooting performance in basketball players. *Sport Psychologist, 16*(1), 34-47. https://doi.org/10.1123/tsp.16.1.34

Pates, J., Oliver, R., & Maynard, I. (2001). The effects of hypnosis on flow states and golf-putting performance. *Journal of Applied Sport Psychology, 4*, 341-354. https://doi.org/10.2466/pms.2000.91.3f.1057

Patterson, D. R., & Jensen, M. P. (2003). Hypnosis and clinical pain. *Psychological Bulletin, 129*(4), 495. http://dx.doi.org/10.1037/0033-2909.129.4.495

Patterson, D. R., Jensen, M. P., Wiechman, S. A., & Sharar, S. R. (2010). Virtual reality hypnosis for pain associated with recovery from physical trauma. *International Journal of Clinical and Experimental Hypnosis, 58*(3), 288-300. https://doi.org/10.1080/00207141003760595

Perfect, M. M., & Elkins, G. R. (2010). Cognitive–behavioral therapy and hypnotic relaxation to treat sleep problems in an adolescent with diabetes. *Journal of Clinical Psychology, 66*(11), 1205-1215. https://doi.org/10.1002/jclp.20732

Plotinus. (1991). *The enneads* (J. Dillon, Ed., & S. MacKenna, Trans.). New York, NY: Penguin Classics.

Potter, G. (2004). Intensive therapy: Utilizing hypnosis in the treatment of substance abuse disorders. *American Journal of Clinical Hypnosis, 47*(1), 21-28. https://doi.org/10.1080/00029157.2004.10401472

Psyche. (n.d.). In *Lexico dictionary*. Retrieved from https://www.lexico.com/en/definition/psyche

Rapkin, D. A., Straubing, M., & Holroyd, J. C. (1991). Guided imagery, hypnosis and recovery from head and neck cancer surgery: An exploratory study. *International Journal of Clinical and Experimental Hypnosis, 39*(4), 215-226. https://doi.org/10.1080/00207149108409637

Raz, A., Fan, J., & Posner, M. I. (2005). Hypnotic suggestion reduces conflict in the human brain. *Proceedings of the National Academy of Sciences of the United States of America, 102*(28), 9978-9983. https://doi.org/10.1073/pnas.0503064102

Raz, A., Zephrani, Z. R., Schweizer, H. R., & Marinoff, G. P. (2004). Critique of claims of improved visual acuity after hypnotic suggestion. *Optometry and Vision Science, 81*(11), 872-879. doi:10.1097/01.OPX.0000145032.79975.58

Retief, F. P., & Cilliers, L. (2008). Medical dreams in Graeco-Roman times. *South African Medical Journal, 95*(11), 841.

Rezaeei, M., & Farahian, M. (2015). Subconscious vs. unconscious learning: A short review of the terms. *American Journal of Psychology and Behavioral Sciences, 2*(3), 98-100.

Rhine, J. B. (1946). Hypnotic suggestion in PK tests. *Journal of Parapsychology, 10,* 126-140.

Richardson, J., Smith, J. E., McCall, G., Richardson, A., Pilkington, K., & Kirsch, I. (2007). Hypnosis for nausea and vomiting in cancer chemotherapy: A systematic review of the research evidence. *European Journal of Cancer Care, 16*(5), 402-412. https://doi.org/10.1111/j.1365-2354.2006.00736.x

Ring, K., & Cooper, S. (2008). *Mind sight: Near death and out of body experiences in the blind*. Bloomington, IN: iUniverse.

Robazza, C., & Bortoli, L. (1995). A case study of improved performance in archery using hypnosis. *Perceptual and Motor Skills, 81*(3), 1364-1366. https://doi.org/10.2466/pms.1995.81.3f.1364

Rock, N. L., Shipley, T. E., & Campbell, C. (1969). Hypnosis with untrained, nonvolunteer patients in labor. *International Journal of Clinical and Experimental Hypnosis, 17*(1), 25-36. https://doi.org/10.1080/00207146908407285

Roediger, L., Joris, J., & Lenny, M. (1995). Hypnosis as adjunct therapy in conscious sedation for plastic surgery. *Regional Anesthesia, 20*(2), 145-151.

Rosén, G., Willoch, F., Bartenstein, P., Berner, N., & Røsjø, S. (2001). Neurophysiological processes underlying the phantom limb pain experience and the use of hypnosis in its clinical management: An intensive examination of two patients. *International Journal of Clinical and Experimental Hypnosis, 49*(1), 38-55. https://doi.org/10.1080/00207140108410378

Ross, U. H., Lange, O., Unterrainer, J., & Laszig, R. (2007). Ericksonian hypnosis in tinnitus therapy: Effects of a 28-day inpatient multimodal treatment concept measured by tinnitus-questionnaire and health survey SF-36. *European Archives of Oto-Rhino-Laryngology, 264*(5), 483-488. doi:10.1007/s00405-006-0221-9

Sanders, S. (1976). Mutual group hypnosis as a catalyst in fostering creative problem solving. *American Journal of Clinical Hypnosis, 19*(1), 62-66. https://doi.org/10.1080/00029157.1976.10403834

Sargent, C. L. (1978). Hypnosis as a psi-conducive state: A controlled replication study. *Journal of Parapsychology, 42*(4), 257.

Schlesinger, I., Benyakov, O., Erikh, I., Suraiya, S., & Schiller, Y. (2009). Parkinson's disease tremor is diminished with relaxation guided imagery. *Movement Disorders, 24*(14), 2059-2062. https://doi.org/10.1002/mds.22671

Schoen, M., & Nowack, K. (2013). Reconditioning the stress response with hypnosis CD reduces the inflammatory cytokine IL-6 and influences resilience: A pilot study. *Complementary Therapies in Clinical Practice, 19*(2), 83-88. https://doi.org/10.1016/j.ctcp.2012.12.004

Schoenberger, N. E., Kirsch, I., Gearan, P., Montgomery, G., & Pastyrnak, S. L. (1998). Hypnotic enhancement of a cognitive behavioral treatment for public speaking anxiety. *Behavior Therapy, 28*(1), 127-140. https://doi.org/10.1016/S0005-7894(97)80038-X

Schreiber, E. H. (1997). Use of group hypnosis to improve college students' achievement. *Psychological Reports, 80*(2), 636-638. https://doi.org/10.2466/pr0.1997.80.2.636

Sharf, R. S. (2012). *Theories of psychotherapy and counseling.* Belmont, CA: Brooks/Cole.

Sheehan, E. P., Smith, H. V., & Forrest, D. W. (1982). A signal detection study of the effects of suggested improvement on the monocular visual acuity of myopes. *International journal of Clinical and Experimental Hypnosis, 30*(2), 138-146. https://doi.org/10.1080/00207148208407379

Sheldrake, R. (2012). *The presence of the past: Morphic resonance and the memory of nature* (2nd ed.). Rochester, VT: Park Street Press.

Siegel, B. S. (1998). *Love, medicine and miracles. Lessons learned about self-healing from a surgeon's experience with exceptional patients* (Reissue ed.). New York, NY: William Morrow Paperbacks.

Sokel, B., Christie, D., Kent, A., & Lansdown, R. (1993). A comparison of hypnotherapy and biofeedback in the treatment of childhood atopic eczema. *Contemporary Hypnosis, 10*(3), 145-154.

Spiegel, D. (2013). Hypnosis and pain control. In T. R. Deer, M. S. Leong, A. Buvanendran, V. Gordin, P. S. Kim, S. J. Panchal, & A. L. Ray (Eds.), *Comprehensive treatment of chronic pain by medical, interventional, and integrative approaches. The American Academy of Pain Medicine textbook on pain management* (pp. 859-866). New York, NY: Springer.

Stanford, R. G., & Stein, A. G. (1994). A meta-analysis of ESP studies contrasting hypnosis and a comparison condition. *Journal of Parapsychology, 58*(3), 235-269.

Sub- prefix. (n.d.). In *Merriam-Webster's online dictionary*. Retrieved from https://www.merriam-webster.com/dictionary/sub

Swirsky-Sacchetti, T., & Margolis, C. G. (1986). The effects of a comprehensive self-hypnosis training program on the use of Factor VIII in severe hemophilia. *International Journal of Clinical and Experimental Hypnosis, 34*(2), 71-83. https://doi.org/10.1080/00207148608406973

Syrjala, K. L., Cummings, C., & Donaldson, G. W. (1992). Hypnosis or cognitive behavioral training for the reduction of pain and nausea during cancer treatment: A controlled clinical trial. *Pain, 48*(2), 137-146. https://doi.org/10.1016/0304-3959(92)90049-H

Tabachnick, B. G., & Fidell, L. S. (2013). *Using multivariate statistics.* Boston, MA: Pearson.

Talbot, M. (1991). *The holographic universe.* New York, NY: Harper Collins.

Tan, G., Fukui, T., Jensen, M. P., Thornby, J., & Waldman, K. L. (2009). Hypnosis treatment for chronic low back pain. *International Journal of Clinical and Experimental Hypnosis, 58*(1), 53-68. https://doi.org/10.1080/00207140903310824

Tart, C. T. (1970). Transpersonal potentialities of deep hypnosis. *Transpersonal Psychology, 2*(1), 27-40.

Tausk, F., & Whitmore, S. E. (1999). A pilot study of hypnosis in the treatment of patients with psoriasis. *Psychotherapy and Psychosomatics, 68*(4), 221-225. https://doi.org/10.1159/000012336

Teeley, A. M., Soltani, M., Wiechman, S. A., Jensen, M. P., Sharar, S. R., & Patterson, D. R. (2012). Virtual reality hypnosis pain control in the treatment of multiple fractures: A case series 1. *American Journal of Clinical Hypnosis, 54*(3), 184-194. https://doi.org/10.1080/00029157.2011.619593

Tressoldi, P., & Del Prete, G. (2007). ESP under hypnosis: The role of induction instructions and personality characteristics. *Journal of Parapsychology, 71*(1), 125-137.

Tressoldi, P. E., Pederzoli, L., Caini, P., Ferrini, A., Melloni, S., Prati, E., & Trabucco, A. (2015). Hypnotically induced out-of-body experience: How many bodies are there? Unexpected discoveries about the subtle body and psychic body. *SAGE Open, Oct.-Dec.,* 1-11. doi:10.1177/2158244015615919

Un- prefix. (n.d.). In *Merriam-Webster's online dictionary*. Retrieved from https://www.merriam-webster.com/dictionary/UN

Vandenbergh, R. L., Sussman, K. E., & Titus, C. C. (1966). Effects of hypnotically induced acute emotional stress on carbohydrate and lipid metabolism in patients with diabetes mellitus. *Psychosomatic Medicine, 4*, 382-390. doi:10.1097/00006842-196607000-00010

Velloso, L. G., Duprat, M. D., Martins, R., & Scoppetta, L. (2010). Hypnosis for management of claustrophobia in magnetic resonance imaging. *Radiologia Brasileira, 43*(1), 19-22. http://dx.doi.org/10.1590/S0100-39842010000100007

Volpe, E. G., & Nash, M. R. (2012). The use of hypnosis for airplane phobia with an obsessive character a case study. *Clinical Case Studies, 11*(2), 89-103. https://doi.org/10.1177/1534650112440167

Wain, H. J., Amen, D., & Jabbari, B. (1990). The effects of hypnosis on a parkinsonian tremor: Case report with polygraph/EEG recordings. *American Journal of Clinical Hypnosis, 33*(2), 94-98. https://doi.org/10.1080/00029157.1990.10402910

Weinstein, E. J., & Au, P. K. (1991). Use of hypnosis before and during angioplasty. *American Journal of Clinical Hypnosis, 34*(1), 29-37. https://doi.org/10.1080/00029157.1991.10402957

Wik, G., Fischer, H., Bragée, B., Finer, B., & Fredrikson, M. (1999). Functional anatomy of hypnotic analgesia: A PET study of patients with fibromyalgia. *European Journal of Pain, 3*(1), 7-12. https://doi.org/10.1016/S1090-3801(99)90183-0

Willemsen, R., Vanderlinden, J., Deconinck, A., & Roseeuw, D. (2006). Hypnotherapeutic management of alopecia areata. *Journal of the American Academy of Dermatology, 55*(2), 233-237. https://doi.org/10.1016/j.jaad.2005.09.025

Williams, J. D., & Gruzelier, J. H. (2001). Differentiation of hypnosis and relaxation by analysis of narrow band theta and alpha frequencies. *International Journal of Clinical and Experimental Hypnosis, 49*(3), 185-206. https://doi.org/10.1080/00207140108410070

Wood, G. J., Bughi, S., Morrison, J., Tanavoli, S., Tanavoli, S., & Zadeh, H. H. (2003). Hypnosis, differential expression of cytokines by T-cell subsets, and the hypothalamo-pituitary-adrenal axis. *American Journal of Clinical Hypnosis, 45*(3), 179-196. https://doi.org/10.1080/00029157.2003.10403525

Xu, Y., & Cardeña, E. (2007). Hypnosis as an adjunct therapy in the management of diabetes. *International Journal of Clinical and Experimental Hypnosis, 56*(1), 63-72. https://doi.org/10.1080/00207140701673050

Yapko, M. D. (1993). Hypnosis and depression. *Handbook of Clinical Hypnosis*, 339-355. http://dx.doi.org/10.1037/10274-016

Yapko, M. D. (2010a). Hypnosis in the treatment of depression: An overdue approach for encouraging skillful mood management. *International Journal of Clinical and Experimental Hypnosis, 58*(2), 137-146. doi:10.1080/00207140903523137

Yapko, M. D. (2010b). Hypnotically catalyzing experiential learning across treatments for depression: Actions can speak louder than moods. *International Journal of Clinical and Experimental Hypnosis, 58*(2), 186-201. https://doi.org/10.1080/00207140903523228

Yexley, M. J. (2007). Treating postpartum depression with hypnosis: Addressing specific symptoms presented by the client. *American Journal of Clinical Hypnosis, 49*(3), 219-223. https://doi.org/10.1080/00029157.2007.10401584

Zachariae, R., Bjerring, P., & Arendt-Nielsen, L. (1989). Modulation of type I immediate and type IV delayed immunoreactivity using direct suggestion and guided imagery during hypnosis. *Allergy, 44*(8), 537-542. https://doi.org/10.1111/j.1398-9995.1989.tb04198.x

Zeltzer, L., Dash, J., & Holland, J. P. (1979). Hypnotically induced pain control in sickle cell anemia. *Pediatrics, 64*(4), 533-536.

Appendix A: Informed Consent

To the Participant in this dissertation research:

You are invited to participate in a study to measure the effect of hypnotic depth and posthypnotic suggestion and visual improvement. This study will be conducted at a private office conference room. This study is being conducted in order to increase the understanding of the effect of hypnosis on visual improvement. By participating in this study, you will be adding to the current literature on hypnosis and visual improvement. You may personally benefit by discovering hidden or latent potentiality that may reside within you. Your participation may also benefit researchers in the area of hypnosis research and vision research as well as expanding our understanding of human potential. Participation is entirely voluntary and that no pressure has been applied to encourage participation.

You will be asked to take part in a hypnosis session where you will be taken in and out of hypnosis a few times and will be asked to read an eye chart before and after posthypnotic suggestion. Deception and misdirection may be used in this study. Posthypnotic suggestions may include the use of temporary conscious amnesia to the suggestion and task at hand. You are aware of and understand that in some cases it may be necessary for the practitioner to respectfully touch your shoulder(s), hand, wrist, or forehead in order to assist you in relaxation. You give the practitioner permission and consent to do so in order to help you establish a beneficial state of hypnosis

Your personal information will be kept strictly confidential. The original data including identifiable information will only be seen by the researcher (Joseph Sansone). Any digital data will be saved in a confidential manner and protected. The hard drive and any printouts of the data will be locked in my office. In addition, peer-reviewers who peruse portions of the work in order to provide an external check to the research will be asked to sign a statement of their agreement to preserve confidentiality. This may include academics and statisticians to help analyze data.

For the protection of your privacy, all information received from you will be kept confidential as to source. Your identity will be protected and identifiable information will not be used in the study. In reporting the findings from this study, any information that might identify you will be altered to insure your anonymity. Though every possible measure will be taken to ensure confidentiality, no online data collection and transmission is 100% secure.

The data from this study may be used for the completion of PhD dissertation research, for publication purposes in academic journals as well as any future books or articles by the researcher (Joseph Sansone). Such publications will exclude all identifiable information.

This study is designed to minimize potential mental distress. While no therapy will be conducted in this research in the rare event that a mental health issue should arise the researcher is qualified to address it and will utilize grounding techniques to stabilize participant and conduct a mental status examination and provide mental health resources such as local therapist information or assist with obtaining more urgent care if needed. If at any time you have any concerns or questions, I, the researcher (Joseph Sansone), will make every effort to discuss them with you and inform you of options for resolving your concerns. You have the right to discontinue participation in this research at any time. The participant may withdraw from the study at any time without penalty or prejudice. Ethical issues please contact the ethics committee below. If you have any questions or concerns, you may call or email:

Joseph Sansone, M.S., LMHC, CCMHC (Researcher)
xxx-xxx-xxxx
joe@xxx.com

Marilyn Schlitz, Ph.D.
Dissertation Committee Chairperson
Sofia University
(650) 493-4430
marilyn.schlitz@sofia.edu

Dr. Frederic Luskin, Ph.D.
Chairperson, Sofia University Research Ethics Committee
(650) 493-4430
cfred.luskin@sofia.edu
1069 East Meadow Circle
Palo Alto, CA 94303 USA

If you decide to participate in this research, you may withdraw your consent and discontinue your participation at any time for any reason without penalty or prejudice. By signing participant acknowledges that the researcher has explained the study to the participant and answered his or her questions. You may request a summary of the research findings which will be a general explanation of the study and results, but with greater explanation, by providing your email address in the space provided on the next page. Such a request will need to be made while research is still being conducted.

_____

Participant's Name (Please print your full legal name)

_____   _____

Participant's Signature   Date

_____   _____

Researcher's Signature   Date

Appendix B: Questionnaire

First Name _____ Last Name _____

Address _____

Phone _____ Email _____

Date of birth _____ Race/Ethnicity _____ Sex _____

List any current medical or mental health diagnosis:

_____

Appendix C: Email Solicitation

Participants needed for a hypnosis study examining the level of hypnotic depth and hypnotic suggestion regarding visual improvement. Participants will undergo hypnosis at a private practice office building. For participation in this study, participants will be provided a trigger to practice self-hypnosis, if desired. Your participation in this study is voluntary and participation will be anonymous. This study has been approved by the Research Ethics Committee at Sofia University, Palo Alto California.

For more information please call Joseph Sansone (xxx-xxx-xxxx), a doctoral candidate at the Institute of Transpersonal Psychology at Sofia University.

Appendix D: Chairs in Private Practice Office

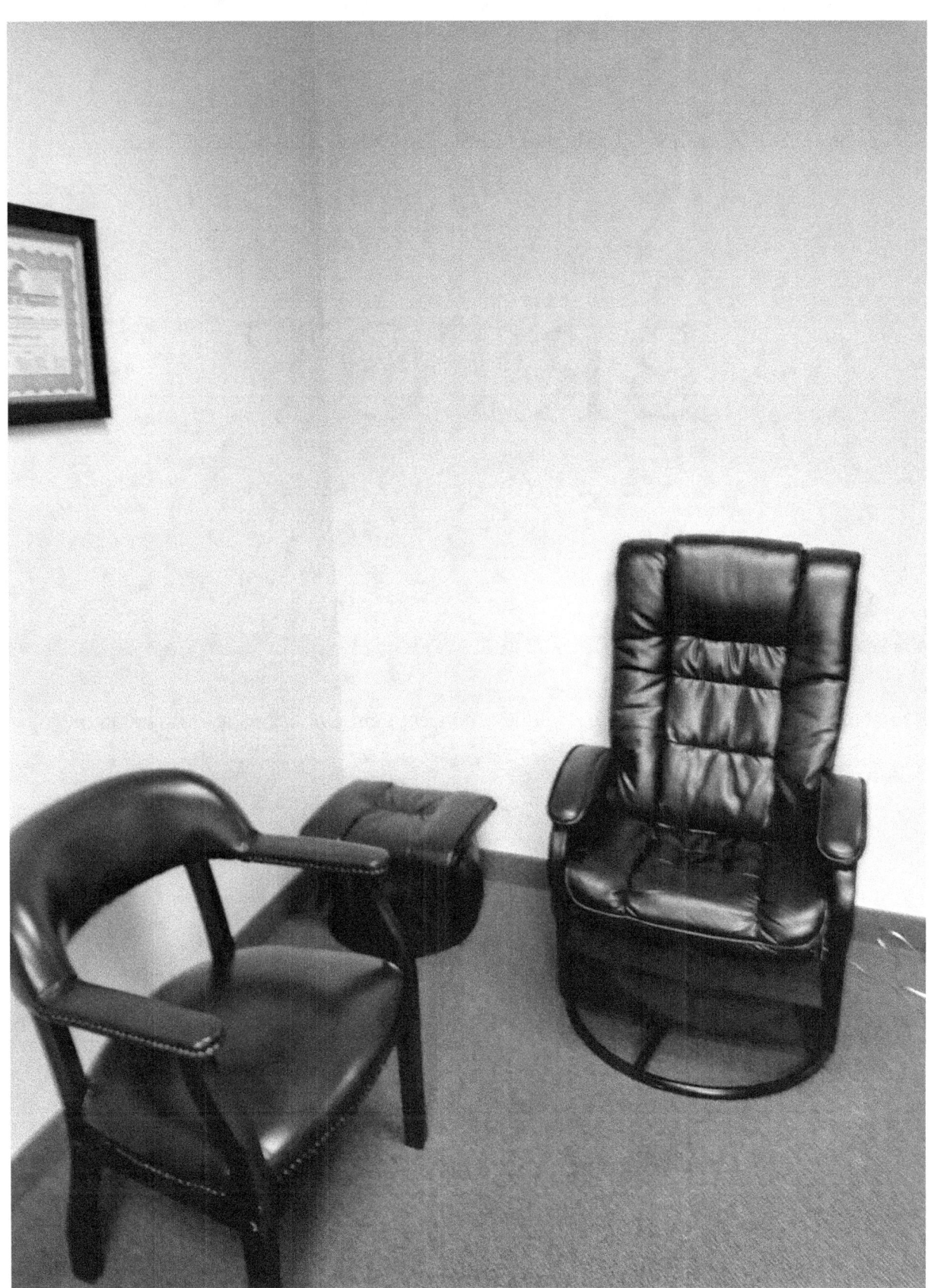

Appendix E: Eye Chart Assessments

Sample of one of 50 variations of a single-line eye chart used in third treatment condition:

BRTOV

The standard eye charts used in first and second treatment conditions are shown on the following two pages.

0.20	O T H V	20/100
0.25	H V T V T	20/80
0.33	V T H O H O	20/60
0.40	T O V T H O V	20/50
0.50	H V O T V O T	20/40
0.66	H V T O T V H	20/30
0.80	V H O T O V H	20/25
1.00	T H V O T V H	20/20
1.25	O H V T H V O	20/16

KASHSURG — 20 FEET EQUIVALENT FOR TESTING AT 10 FEET (3 METERS)

CE

	KASHSURG	20 FEET EQUIVALENT FOR TESTING AT 10 FEET (3 METERS)
0.20	**T Z C O**	20/100
0.25	**L D P O F**	20/80
0.33	**P T O C E T**	20/60
0.40	**Z L P E D T C**	20/50
0.50	**E T O D C F O**	20/40
0.66	D P C Z L F T	20/30
0.80	C F D T E O P	20/25
1.00	L D C Z O T E	20/20
1.25	P F O D T E L	20/16

CE

Appendix F: Eye Chart on Stand

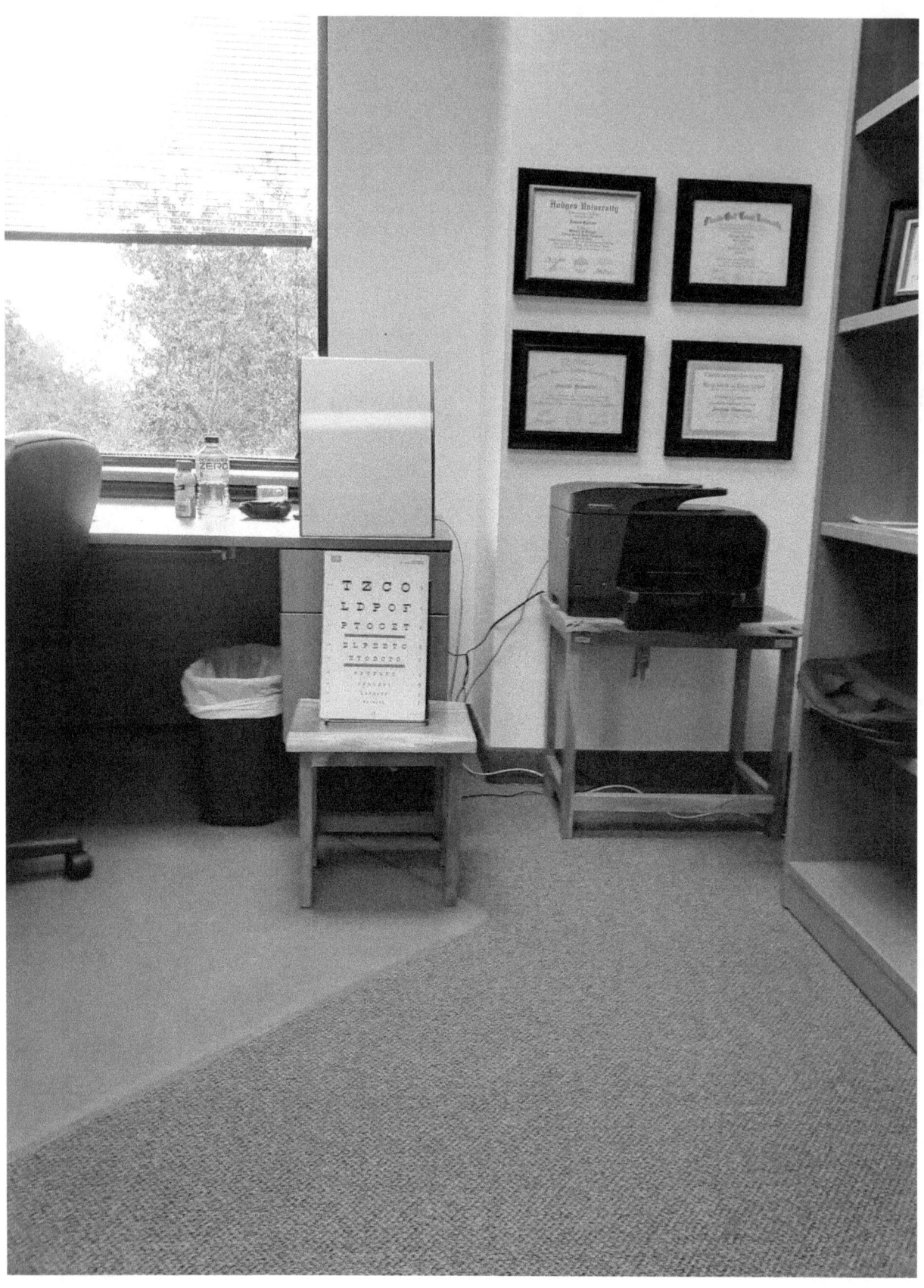

Appendix G: Shielding Eye Chart

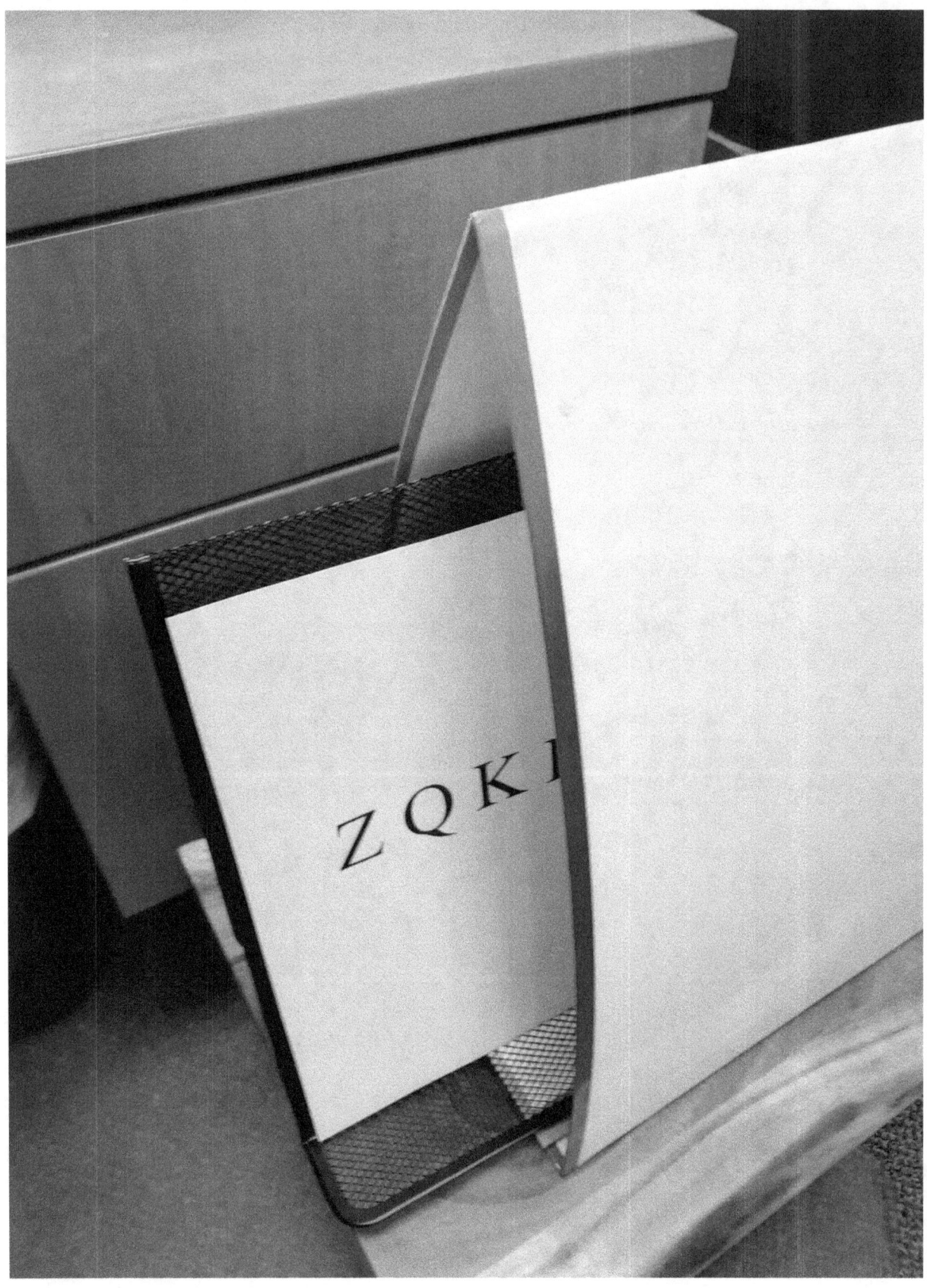

Appendix H: Shielded Eye Chart

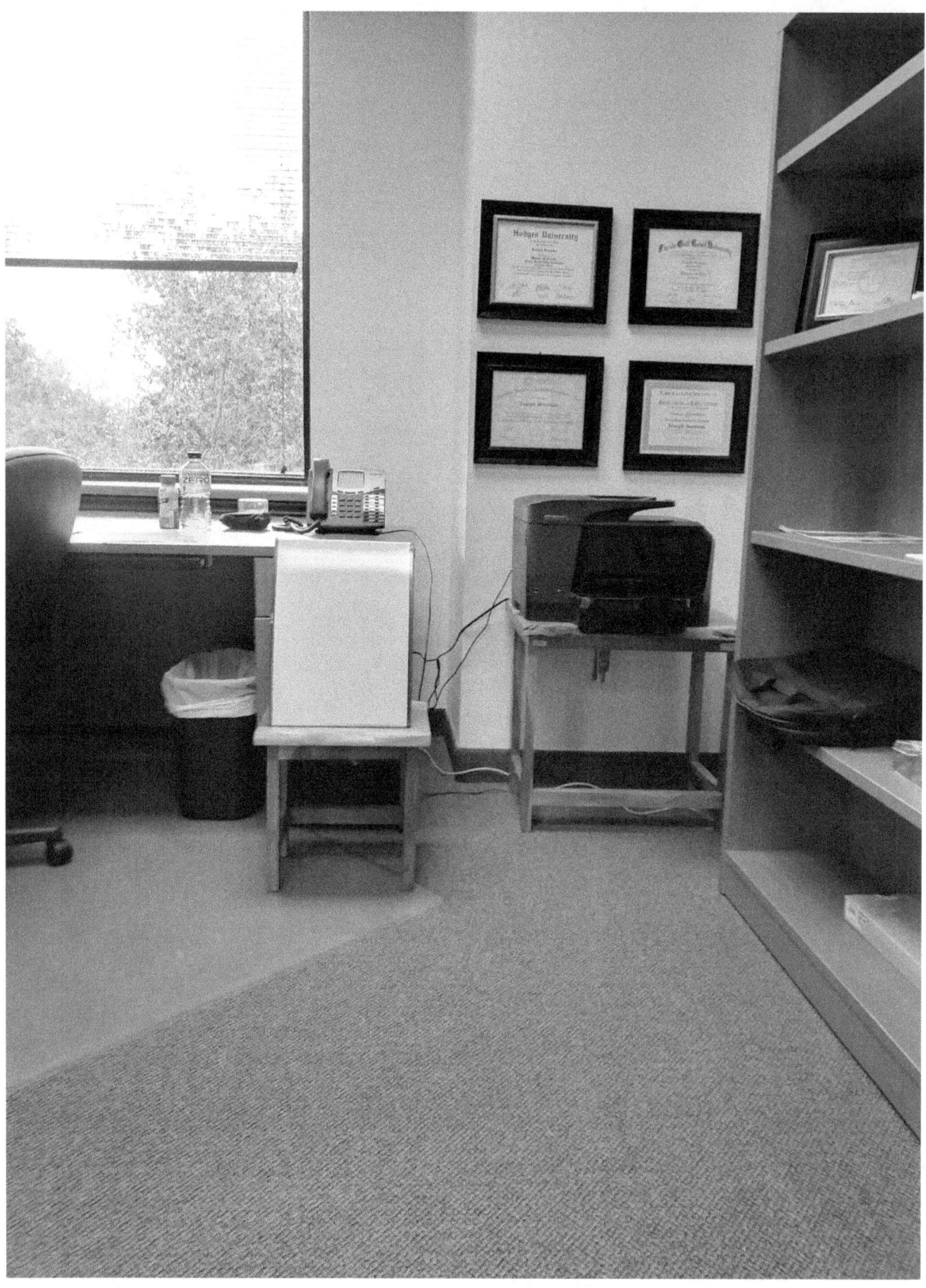

Appendix I: Posthypnotic Suggestion Sample

Sample posthypnotic suggestions for visual improvement:

Your eyes have cellular memory just like you have muscle memory. Your eyes will use that cellular memory and remember back to a time when your vision was effortlessly crystal clear. With your eyes totally relaxed your vision will be crystal clear with laser sharp focus. The contrast will be sharper and the colors more vivid. In a moment when I count from one to three with your eyes totally relaxed you will read the eye chart with laser sharp totally relaxed crystal-clear vision.

Sample posthypnotic suggestion for nonphysical sight:

I am going to give you a powerful posthypnotic suggestion where your conscious mind will not remember the suggestion, but your subconscious mind will remember it and act on it. In a moment, this time when I count from 1 to 3, you will read five letters in a single-line eye chart from left to right. The letters are bigger and easier to read than the previous eye chart. There is a small dry-erase board in front of the eye chart. You will not be able to see the dry-erase board. The dry-erase board will be invisible to you, and your perceptual field will either see through or around the dry-erase board, and read it easily and effortlessly.

www.ingramcontent.com/pod-product-compliance
Lightning Source LLC
Chambersburg PA
CBHW081156290426
44108CB00018B/2569